Gold

A Lifetime of Love
in Chiropractic

DR. IRENE GOLD, DC

DR. JUDD NOGRADY, DC

"The pursuit of knowledge for its own sake, an almost fanatical love of justice, and the desire for personal independence - these are the features of the Jewish tradition which make me thank my stars that I belong to it."
–Albert Einstein

"If you are not out to change the world, everything, else is just Mickey Mouse."
–Reggie Gold

"I am an ordinary person who was able to live an extraordinary life through a commitment to excellence, persistence, and a mission much bigger than myself."

–Irene Gold

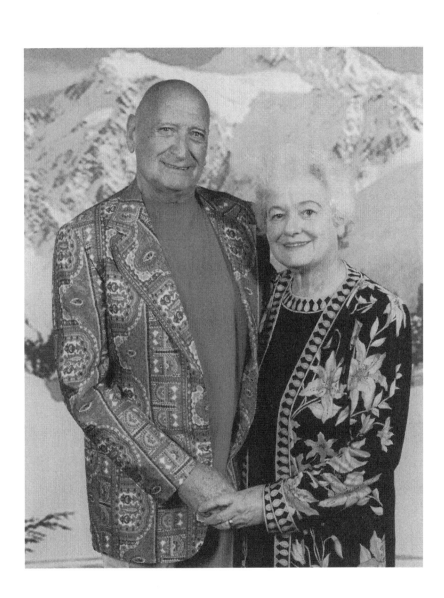

Table of Contents

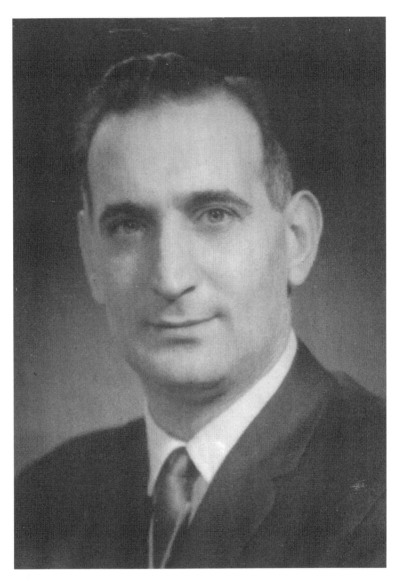

Reggie Gold

Chapter 1

Love

The history of Chiropractic has been shaped by rugged, dynamic pioneers. We have a long history of strong leadership. The most dynamic couple we've ever had in Chiropractic is Reggie and Irene Gold. Irene has taught more Chiropractors than any other person in history. This fact alone is mind-boggling! Irene and her company, Irene Gold Associates, have helped more Chiropractors gain licensure than any other company in the world.

Reggie was a true pioneer. He espoused his ideas about Chiropractic worldwide and advanced a whole new philosophy of Chiropractic. Irene has taught at three Chiropractic colleges and has taught Chiropractors from every college in the world with her board review program.

Whereas B.J. Palmer taught "One Cause, One Cure", Reggie espoused the idea that Chiropractic improved body function regardless of symptoms. He felt deeply that Chiropractic care was for all people, sick or well, because Chiropractic helps the body to function better at all levels.

One can argue or discuss philosophy all night and into the next day, as many Chiropractors do. It can be argued that B.J. taught that the Chiropractic adjustment got man, the human, closer to the Creator; however, it cannot be argued that B.J.'s search in Chiropractic was doing the least to the body and getting the best result. B.J. spent a lifetime locating the cause of dis-ease.

Reggie spent a lifetime inspiring Chiropractors to look beyond tangible results and observe the effect that Chiropractic care has on every level of human potential.

As I interviewed Chiropractors that are close to the Golds, there emerged a clear pattern. Universally, people said that when Reggie spoke, it was as if they understood the depth of Chiropractic for the first time. Many long time practitioners expressed the same sentiment. They didn't speak much around Reggie, they only listened.

Reggie's eloquence as a speaker was unmatched, and his take home message lasted many for a lifetime. Many of the same people said, almost in the same breath, that if it wasn't for Irene, Reggie wouldn't have gotten nearly as far. The same doctors that praised Reggie's oratory skills and great mind stood in agreement that Irene was the real brain. This stands in direct contrast to Irene's statement that Reggie was the smartest man she ever knew, and that next to him, she felt small, as his intellectual power astounded her.

So what and who are the real Irene and Reggie? They had a deep, binding love with each other and with Chiropractic for over fifty years! Their gifts to others will live forever. Reggie immediately seized the why of Chiropractic, while Irene was enthralled with its practical aspects. Her years in nursing led her to look on with amazement as she saw people get better without medications or dietary changes. In her words, "it was amazing that people got better, and all Reggie did was 'merely adjust the atlas.'"

Let's explore the life of the greatest Chiropractic partnership, so we may learn; and as we learn, let us grow; and as we grow let us inspire others.

Chapter 2

Pioneers

A type of mind seems to believe that because all the earth is known and the country is settled, no further pioneering remains to be done.

Thus far, the pioneers have been working outside of things; nowadays, the new direction of pioneering is toward the inside of things. We know the planet pretty well; we are now exploring the atom. We are only in the far off, dim beginnings of knowledge. Discoveries are yet to be made, greater than those of Columbus - but in another region. The youth of today live in a more thrilling period than those of the merchant adventurer or the early frontiersmen.

There are pioneers, plodders or parasites. Pioneers made the venture and conquest. Plodders consolidate the hold that has been gained. Parasites follow and live off others' labors.

Each fulfills a purpose, even the parasite. He is pretty low down on the scale, like the maggot, but his presence is an advertisement that something exists on which he can live. It is likewise a warning that "that something", whatever it may be, should be eliminated.

We cannot afford to view life from the maggot's or parasite's point of view, nor even justify them because they fulfill a scavenger's duty; as human beings, we are bent upon securing a mode of life where these simple things die for want of sustenance. Pioneers are far more interesting, and more worth emphasis.

Most of us would not have to go far back into our families to find a pioneer. There may even be pioneers among our recent newcomers to America, although no longer does any doubt exist that the number and ratio of parasites have increased.

Most of us are here today because some men and women were brave enough to venture across strange lands to make a life as they wanted it.

There is this about the pioneer: he is a man of courage and vision in the community. Timid people stay home. People who live in the rut do not venture far. The pioneer has the vision to see new regions and the spirit to conquer them.

Partial reprint of Palmer Green Book, Volume 32, Chapter 18,
written by Dr. B.J. Palmer, Chiropractor.

Chapter 3

Chiropractic is more than a career, it's a life path

For many, the long, rough, rugged road of being a Chiropractor wears them down. This same rough road sharpened Irene and Reggie Gold to a razor's edge. They found Chiropractic and fully embraced it. They lived a life of service and gratitude toward the profession and "Chiropractic."

We cannot usually separate our beginnings from our becoming; our earliest years seem to somehow shape all our actions for years to come. As time passes we begin to feel comfortable in our new skin. Then we examine our past, and through examining it, we grow.

Irene

My parents were immigrants. My dad was from Germany and my mom was from England. Our family name was Siemens. My mother was an uneducated woman who never attended school past the seventh grade. My father had absolutely no formal education. The only schooling he had was a rudimentary flight school prior to becoming a pilot in World War I, on the German side.

In the early days of aviation it was not uncommon for pilots to have very minimal education. Pilots were often picked by general aptitude, and training was done in a sink or swim method. Many of these early pilots had never seen an airplane, yet training protocol often had them flying within six weeks or less. The loss of life was near 80%, with large numbers of fatalities occurring during training.

My mother came to America around 1909. My father had stowed away on a cargo ship and entered America illegally after the war, sometime around 1921. They met on the lower east side of New York City, at a candy store that my mother's family owned. My mother was an industrious woman who helped run the family business.

When my father first got to America he quickly went to work. He had some wiring skills, most learned from the WWI planes, and he had some mechanical knowledge from the work he did in the service. He quickly became an electrician.

Dad was quite a character. He became self-employed partly because he preferred to work for himself, and mostly because he had strong opinions and convictions.

My parents met in 1928, they were married in 1929. People at that time were not so caught up with big romances, but were more practical. They were two immigrants and they knew if they worked together they could get ahead. They had their first of six children in 1934, and the last was born in 1940. I was the third child and first daughter. For a brief time there were four of us until my oldest brother was killed in a fire when he was just about five. There was a large bonfire on the street, and somehow he fell in and was burned to death.

My folks had us living in a two room apartment, one bedroom and one kitchen/dining room combination. There was a small bathroom off to the side. We spent five years in those two rooms. To say we were a close family was an understatement! This close family bond has lasted a lifetime. I've been extremely fortunate to have a great, loving relationship with all of my siblings.

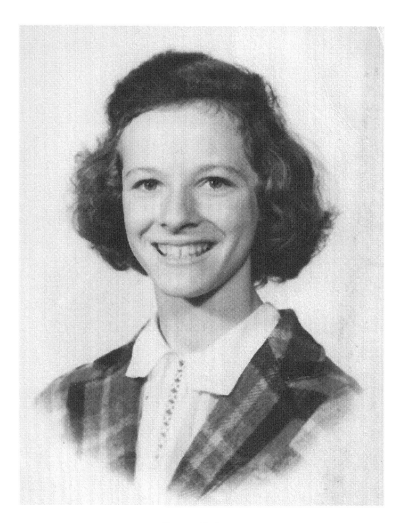

Irene Seimens

Richard, my oldest brother, became an extremely successful land developer in Florida. My younger brother Walter was also a land developer in New York until his untimely death. Marion, my sister, became an extremely accomplished math teacher with a long history of teaching. Carrie, the youngest, is a very successful real-estate broker.

It's interesting to note that one of my family's greatest accomplishments is that we've all had long, successful marriages, and we've all spent a lifetime with our original spouses.

In 1947, we moved out of New York City and settled in Spring Valley, NY. We lived in a house that my father built. He started construction in 1940 and finished it in 1947. He'd first purchased 12 acres of land for $900. My parents were very poor, I mean we had nothing. They saved whatever they could, and that $900 represented a great deal of scrimping and saving.

When we moved in, the house was "finished", which meant it stood upright. We had no plumbing, no electric, and no central heat. All the heat for the entire house came out of a large wood stove in the kitchen. We went to bed with a pile of blankets, which was the only way to avoid freezing on cold nights. All the water for cooking and bathing came from a pump in the side yard. The toilet "outhouse" was in the backyard.

We had chickens, ducks, and a large garden. There was no public transportation to school, so I was enrolled in a yeshiva (a Jewish elementary or secondary school) because they provided bus transportation. When I attended school in the city, I was considered a great student and was placed one year ahead. When I entered my first real school, I realized I'd only been pushed ahead because many of the inner city students did not have an interest in education as a

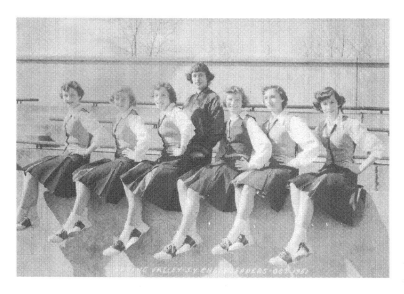

Irene, third from right

Turns to Nursing

IRENE SIEMENS

Plans to Study at Flower Fifth Ave.

Irene Siemens, a member of this year's graduating class of Spring Valley High School, will enter the Flower-Fifth Avenue School of Nursing in New York City next fall, where she will prepare for the nursing profession.

In high school, Irene has been active in girls' intramural sports, for which she won a sports letter. She also won a band letter and a chorus letter for her activity in music. Irene is a member of the German Club, a special privilege student and a member of the School Service Corps. She is treasurer of the senior class and a member of the General Organization Assembly.

Irene is the daughter of Mr. and Mrs. Max Siemens of 1 Union Road, Spring Valley.

priority in their lives. The only reason they were in school was because it was the law.

When I started at the yeshiva they realized I wasn't really ahead, but actually behind, especially in reading. I started the yeshiva school at eleven years old and entered into the seventh grade with two other students. I felt very isolated because the two girls were good friends and I was the odd girl out.

School was very lonely in the beginning. On top of that, my mother and father expected us to be independent from an early age. They didn't accompany us to the school functions or any other outings that most parents attended with children. I always had to travel alone. I think they were trying to help us to become independent, but it was very frightening for me, and I became very shy.

As I slowly met more students and saw how they lived, I realized how poor my family was. I realized that we were the only family in the area that lived the way we did. I remember one night I couldn't go home because of a big snow storm. I went home with a classmate that lived nearby, and it was the first time I'd been in a house with a regular bed and bathroom, and heat! It was shocking to me that people lived so well and stayed warm all night.

As I continued through school, I was trying to figure out what I was going to do with my life. My older brother had a girlfriend that was in nursing school, and she recommended nursing as a good occupation. When I turned sixteen I applied to Flower 5th Ave Hospital School of Nursing. The school was located in Manhattan on 105th St. and 5th Avenue.

I got accepted to the nursing program, but before I could attend class I had to have a physical exam. The trip to the physical took three buses and almost two hours of travelling. The physical was a quick affair, maybe ten

School of Nursing   June 26, 1953

Miss Irene Siemens
1 Union Road
Spring Valley, New York

Dear Miss Siemens:

　　　　　We find that you did not pass our physical
examination due to hypertension.

　　　　　While our health officer feels that this may
not interfere with your nursing, it is our policy that a waiver
must be signed by your parents before we can finally accept you.
We would suggest that you see your family physician.

　　　　　Would you please come in to discuss this matter
at your earliest convenience. You may write, or telephone
TRafalgar 6-5500, Ext. 346 for an appointment.

　　　　　　　　　　　　　　　Sincerely yours,

　　　　　　　　　　　　　　　Helen M. Daum
　　　　　　　　　　　　　　　Director of Nursing

HMD:ljs

minutes, and then I was dismissed and told to go home. About four weeks later an envelope arrived in the mail. It stated that I would not be allowed to attend nursing school because I failed the physical due to high blood pressure. There was an option, which of course I took, to sign a waiver that if I died, my family couldn't sue the school.

I would start nursing school in the fall, and this would be the first time I'd be away from my family. My parents had their shortcomings, as all parents do, but they thought their children were the finest children in the world, and their pride in us was palpable. They instilled in us a desire to get an education and work hard. All five children went to college and two got advanced degrees. We all went to work.

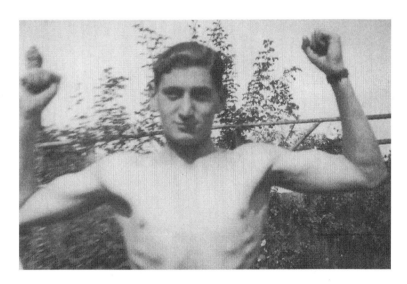

Reggie showing off his buff body!

Chapter 4

The cream always rises to the top!

Reggie

Reggie was born in Europe in December, 1925, and grew up in a very poor section of London. Some thought his parents were a mismatch. His father was a very rough man while his mother was known as the gentlest of ladies. She had an eloquence that surrounded her, and it was with she that Reggie bonded. Reggie never spoke much of his relationship with his father, but it was generally known that they didn't get on well. He and Reggie never saw things the same way, and they had a very poor relationship in general. Reggie had three siblings, a sister Lee, a brother Jack (now deceased), and a younger brother Martin. When Martin was in his late teens he committed suicide. How this early suicide affected Reggie is unknown because he never discussed it.

When Reggie started primary school he immediately ran into problems. It was discovered that he was intellectually gifted, and there wasn't much the school could teach him, as he quickly outgrew the educational requirements of the day. He had more facts and questions than anyone could answer or account for. It was quickly decided that school was no place for him.

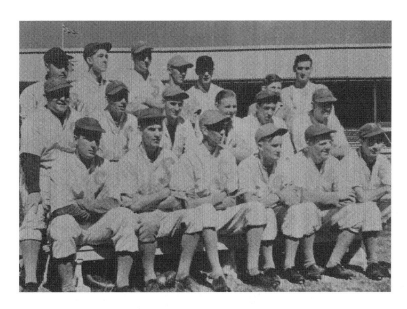

Reggie (back row on right) was a super athlete and he excelled in baseball.

At that time period an advanced education was not considered to be a real advantage in life. He was a young boy growing up in pre-World War II London. It was a world marked by global depression and war. As a young boy growing up at such a time, there were many more things considered much more important than a formal education. Like many youngsters from his area, he went to work at an early age, and helped in the family candy making business.

One thing that separated Reggie from many of his peers was religion. Being a Jew could be a real isolator. Anti-Semitism was common, and being a Jew in pre-World War II Europe could be a lonely and frightening experience. Reggie was instructed in the fundamentals of the Jewish religion and had a Bar Mitzvah* at the age of thirteen. Being a Jew certainly prepared Reggie in terms of being an underdog, always looking for a fair shake or a fight.

As soon as age allowed, he joined the military. As in many aspects of life in Europe, there was strong anti-Semitism in the British military. Because of his lack of formal education, Reggie was put into basic training. They say cream always rises to the top, and in Reggie's case, he couldn't help but rise. His natural intelligence and determination were quickly noticed, and he was promoted to officer's training.

It wasn't just intelligence that distinguished Reggie, but his drive, and an intense desire to be the best, that got him noticed. Reggie became a British officer, but because of his religion, he never quite fit in with his fellow officers. Despite the hardships imposed by isolation, Reggie loved military life, and had every intention of becoming a military man and making it his career. It seems strange that a free thinker would enjoy the drills and monotony of military life, but Reggie saw the military as a higher service. It was a calling.

While serving in Syria, he became involved in an operation to smuggle guns to Jews living in Palestine. As Reggie tells the story, "It's no secret that I am Jewish. In the early Arab-Israeli conflicts, my sympathies were obviously with the Israelis. Even if I had not been directly involved through ethnic ties, I just like the underdog in a fight. I got involved with running guns to Israel. We had a lot of captured German and Italian weapons. The Arab

---

* Bar Mitzvah the religious initiation ceremony of a Jewish boy who has reached the age of 13 and is regarded as ready to observe religious precepts.

armies outnumbered the Israelis about 300 to 1. We thought we would even up the odds a little. I say 'we' because there was a group of British officers involved, very few of whom were Jewish, incidentally. I got caught by the Egyptian police while we were crossing the border at a place called Kantara, and was taken to Port Said. I was beaten up pretty badly and sentenced to life in prison."

No one can be sentenced to "life" without some effect on their mental psyche. As Reggie said, "it was quite a shock."

When Reggie made friends, they often stuck by very closely. Often times, these grew into lifelong friendships. When he was in the service he made such a friend, and this particular friend had contacts throughout the government. He quickly bribed and bartered for Reggie's freedom. As a result, Reggie was released and quickly reclaimed by the British army.

In 1948, Reggie came to the realization that military life was not in his future. He discovered that after the war, promotions came in ten year increments, and his religion would further hamper that slow upward movement. Reggie left the service as the youngest major in the entire British army. But when Reggie got home as a civilian, he found the fight wasn't over.

"It seemed I couldn't get away from a fight. When I got home from the war there were British Fascist groups in London who liked to march through the streets, find a Jew alone, and beat him up or throw him through a store window. I joined a group called G3, which was an underground group of 43 Jewish ex-servicemen who didn't want to see Fascism get established back in England."

"When I joined this group, I began promoting it as part of a speakers group. That's how I got my very first

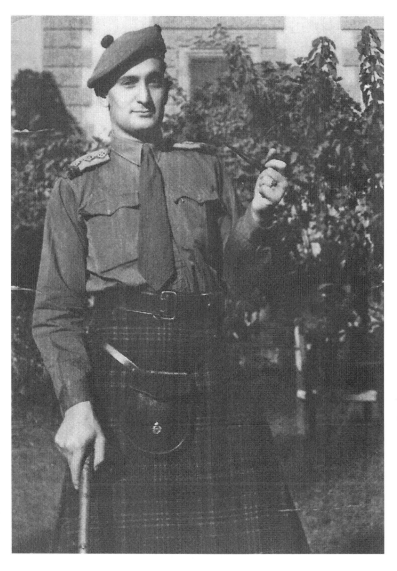

Reggie was a British paratrooper and combat veteran of WWII. He held the rank of major, and was the youngest major in the British armed forces.

experience as a public speaker - on a soap box in Hyde Park, making the public aware of what was going on."

In 1948, Reggie and his entire family immigrated to the United States. Quite by accident Reggie ran into an old schoolmate and they went into the antique business. This business took off rapidly, and it allowed Reggie to travel and use his mind. There was so much to learn about antiques. It seemed that he'd found the perfect business.

As Reggie traveled the world buying and selling antiques, he would think, "this is a great way to make a living, but I want more from life. I want to do something that makes a difference." Little did he know that his life calling would find him.

As has happened with many others before him, an illness in the form of unrelenting asthma brought Reggie into contact with Chiropractic. When he moved to the States, Reggie became a severe asthmatic. A friend told Reggie, "You may think I'm crazy, but why don't you see a Chiropractor?"

At this time there was no licensure, and you could only get an appointment with a Chiropractor through patient referral. When new patients got to the office they had to pass the "who sent you?" test. It was common to undergo a question and answer test before you could even get in the door.

Early Chiropractors had to be extremely careful about accepting new patients, because new people were often plants sent to entrap early practitioners for practicing "medicine" without a license. It is testament to the early practitioner of Chiropractic that Chiropractic not only survived, but actually increased during this period.

Early practices were completely patient driven. People got well with Chiropractic care and spread the word to family, friends, and neighbors about the wonders of the new and growing science of "Chiropractic." These fiercely loyal clients, many of whom owed their life to Chiropractic care, felt they owed a debt to humanity. Most of these people had been written off by medical doctors, and when they returned to their family M.D. with their "Chiropractic story", they were told Chiropractic was a hoax, or worse. However, people like these became determined that Chiropractic had to survive.

Reggie's first visit to Dr. Frank Peruso was a real eye-opener for him. The concepts explained just clicked. Initially, Reggie didn't experience results from care. But as he talked to people in the waiting room, one person after another told him of the great results they were getting, and he became more interested.

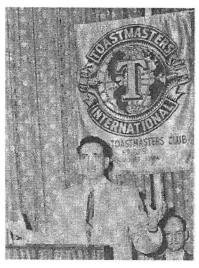

TOASTMASTERS CONTEST

In true traditional Toastmastering style, Palmer's most promising Toastmaster, Reg Gold, emerged victorious for the second straight year in the annual Toastmasters District 19 Speech Contest held at Des Moines, Iowa on May 4th.

Reg had previously qualified for this honor by placing first on the individual club level and then in the Area 4 Contest. He was one of seven participants representing 1250-1300 Toastmasters throughout the State of Iowa and part of Illinois. Next he shall represent Iowa on the Zone level against five other states. This year the Zone Conference is to be held at Davenport. The contest winner there will proceed to Dallas, Texas for the International Speech Contest and final honors.

Reggie belonged to the Toastmasters Club 1917. He won two consecutive Toastmaster District annual speech contests.

His mother had suffered seven strokes, and medical care had not helped her in the slightest. He wondered if this "new" form of care could help her. He brought her to the office where she was adjusted, upper cervical on a side posture table, atlas only. She received tremendous results from Chiropractic care, and Reggie was impressed!

By now, he was so taken with Chiropractic that he began to read everything he could get his hands on. Much of what he read was written by B.J. Palmer, so naturally Reggie went to Palmer. In order to be admitted to Palmer back then you had to have a high school degree, which Reggie didn't have, so he had to take a High School equivalency entrance exam.

Like many other students, Reggie had to work full time in order to pay his way through Palmer. He worked 30 to 40 hour weeks while attending school. Reggie held many interesting positions, which varied from selling anything and everything as a door to door salesman, to being a museum curator, and doing radio shows.

In addition to working long hours, Reggie was class president, valedictorian, and student representative for International Chiropractors Association (ICA). He was also in the Toastmaster speakers club and won many public speaking contests in the Midwest.

These accomplishments are tremendous for any student, but they are especially impressive when you look at some of Reggie's classmates. These included Joe Flesia, who went on to run Renaissance Seminars with Guy Reikeman, President of Life University, and Jerry McAndrews, who became the director of the ICA. Other notable students who were at Palmer while Reggie was there included Sid Williams (founder of Life College), Thom Gelardi (Founder of Sherman College), John Miller (President of

Palmer West), and Chuck Gibson, who still runs a very successful Chiropractic seminar business.

21

Reggie was totally engrossed in and fascinated with Chiropractic, especially the philosophy of Chiropractic. His philosophy instructor was Galen Price. Reggie could spend hours discussing or reading Chiropractic philosophy, and he couldn't understand why other students weren't as fascinated with it as he was.

Not all teachers at Palmer were as interesting and committed as Dr. Price. There was one instructor whose main function, it seemed, was putting students down and making their lives miserable. This particular instructor had a special fondness for picking on one particularly humble student. During one class, the professor called this student "an obstetrical accident", and that was too much for Reggie to put up with. He got up in class and challenged the instructor both mentally and physically. As tempers flared, Reggie suddenly turned and left. He went straight to B.J. Palmer. He protested against the treatment handed out by this instructor, not for himself, but towards his fellow students. He argued so eloquently that B.J. fired this instructor on the spot.

After that the students were all for Reggie, he'd earned a place in their hearts! Years later, Irene received a letter from the student who'd been the object of ridicule by this particular instructor. In his letter, he explained to Irene just what kind of person Reggie was, and how Reggie had saved him. He'd been on the verge of quitting Palmer before Reggie stood up for him. He further explained that he'd gone on to have a successful practice and family life, and he felt he owed it all to Reggie.

When Reggie was at Palmer, B.J. was respected and revered. As Reggie matured, he looked back at his time at Palmer. He was always wishful that he could have talked to B.J. more, and discussed with him his new ideas for Chiropractic. Reggie felt that B.J., who was always open to discussing new ideas about Chiropractic, would have agreed that the natural progression of Chiropractic was in the direction towards Reggie's new philosophy, and the concept that Chiropractic is for the improvement of human potential.

Chapter 5

We all have to start "somewhere!"

Irene

My family had absolutely no money, so in order for us to survive we all worked. I'd always worked around the house since as far back as I could remember, but I got my first job earning money at 13. I have many great memories of my childhood, but my family was always one step away from catastrophe.

At that time women were thought of as inferior to men, and my brothers got more attention. It's hard to explain, but somehow males at that time were regarded as full people, while women were regarded as somewhat less. We were expected to contribute and work, but not many people were interested in our opinion. What we thought didn't seem to matter much.

My younger brother Walter, whom I was closest with, got rheumatic fever when he was young. When he was 15 years old he was diagnosed with subacute bacterial endocarditis. He battled his entire life. A public health nurse visited the house to explain future care, which included taking antibiotics daily. This visit led to my pursuing a career as a public health nurse.

When Walter was 28 years old, he was badly burned in a gas explosion. He had many surgeries and everyone thought he would die. When I visited him in the hospital after the accident, I couldn't even recognize him due to his injuries.

He finally managed to get out of the hospital, but he had a very difficult time breathing. Later, in an effort to try to breathe more easily, he agreed to have open heart surgery. The surgery was somewhat successful and it allowed him to live until the age of 64. At this time he needed to undergo another surgery, which killed him. I am proud that all three of his children have gone to college and became successful, and I am equally proud that all of his children and grandchildren have been under Chiropractic care.

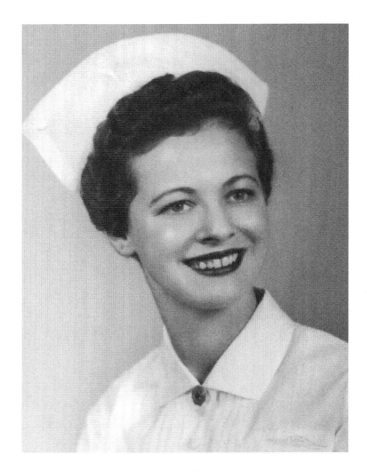

Irene Siemens

Chapter 6

Off to school

On the first day of nursing school, 63 women showed up. I paid $525 for nursing school, which was three years tuition in advance, and included room and board. My father agreed to send me one dollar a week for which I was grateful. Bus fare home was a $1.06, so I settled in, and learned how to stretch that dollar.

While attending nursing school I was required to work in the hospital without pay. I would take care of 35 patients on the overnight shift. In the hospital we sometimes received tips. I didn't work for the tips, but because I'd been raised to always do my absolute best, and because I truly loved people, I received a lot of tips. As I made money I would send half to my brother, and then save some, spending as little as possible because that was how we were raised. Always save as much as possible because rainy days were inevitable.

In the hospital where I worked there were many people who were in oxygen tents, as well as people with IV's and tons of diseases. Many of these cases were terminal. I was 19 years old and in charge of the entire ward. I got a tremendous education, but it was trial by fire. We received lots of practical experience and had excellent classes. I got a good education. When I graduated with my RN degree, I decided to become a public health nurse.

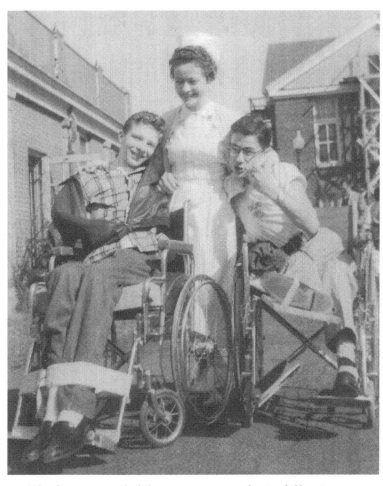

*The boy on my left became a paraplegic following an
immunization and spent the rest of his life in a wheelchair.*

A public health nurse is a nurse that goes into peoples' homes and helps with various things, from colostomy bags to helping new mothers with child care. In order to be accepted into the home nursing program, I needed six months of experience, and I couldn't begin the program for six months. I spent the first two months in a regular hospital and found out quickly that it wasn't the type of work for me.

I spent the next four months working in a rehab hospital. Most of the time I was assigned to patients aged 16 years and older who were paraplegics and quadriplegics. My time working with these brave young people put life into perspective. If you can walk and feed yourself, you are doing well, never mind all the comforts.

I received a stipend from New York State to obtain my certificate in public health nursing. I spent one year at the University of Pennsylvania getting that certificate, and then I went to Columbia University, and spent two more years to finish my bachelor's degree while working full time as a public health nurse.

I decided to switch to school nursing and spent the next eight years at Columbia University, taking evening and summer classes to get my master's degree in health education, while working full time at the Tappan elementary school as a school nurse.

After getting the master's, I enrolled at NYU in order to attain a PhD in school administration. I never finished that degree because I went to Chiropractic college instead.

Chapter 7

A matchmakers dream

Irene and Reggie - 1958-60

I was working as a traveling public health nurse. I liked being in touch with people, going directly into their homes, because it gave me a special bond with people. The pay was good and it was regular nine to five hours with weekends off. Reggie graduated from Palmer in 1957, and in early 1958 he went home to his family in New Jersey. Because Palmer College was not accredited in New Jersey when he graduated, he went looking for an office in nearby New York State.

In 1951, before he started college, Reggie bought himself a new car. It was a 1951 Cadillac Series 61 four door, but by 1958 it had begun to show its age, and was well worn since his student days at Palmer. While on a trip looking for a place to practice, his car broke down and he found himself in Spring Valley, NY.

As Reggie looked around and waited for his car to be repaired, he began to like the look of Spring Valley. There was an insurance office on the corner and Reggie stopped in. During the conversation the insurance agent let on that he didn't need all the office space he had, so he offered to split his office with Reggie. Reggie jumped at the chance, but he probably got the worst office layout in history. The office was laid out like a bowling alley, about 8 feet wide by 40 feet long, and L-shaped at that.

The only thing holding up the deal was money. Reggie's family was in no position to lend him money, so his first stop was a Chiropractor that he had met at Lyceum. Reggie knew he ran a very successful office in Pearl River, New York. When Reggie got to Pearl River, he laid out his plan and his promise to repay. Much to his surprise, the Chiropractor, Dr. Gerhardt Pepper, reached into his pocket and gave Reggie a $700 loan on the spot! It was a generous offer and it got Reggie started.

Reggie knew he had to start getting people in the door, so he went back to what he knew best, which was speaking. His first stop was to the local synagogue. He asked the Rabbi if there was a youth group he could join. The Rabbi informed Reggie that there wasn't a youth group in Spring Valley, but by sheer coincidence there'd been another young man inquiring about exactly the same thing just a few days earlier. (Sheer coincidences seem to pile up when you are on the right track in life). The Rabbi proposed that if Reggie and this young man would set up a youth group, they could use the synagogue for their meeting. He also sweetened the deal by providing a list of all the single young people in the community.

As Reggie's philosophy grew, his religious ideals changed. He always loved the Jewish culture, but he began to disagree with the dogma of any religion. Reggie was a spiritualist. He believed that the same energy that animated the universe also brought life into the body. He felt that when our time here on earth was over, that the energy must go somewhere. He knew that the world was animated in such a wonderful and fantastic way that it could not all be mere chance. Reggie could not accept all the rules that religions imposed in order to be accepted.

Spring Valley was my town. I was working as a public health nurse, and I spent weekends working in the local hospital. I knew practically everyone. When the new youth group started up, I heard about it through the synagogue. One evening while at the synagogue, I went to look into this new group. As Reggie spoke, I began to think, "He's a doctor, I'm a nurse, maybe we have something in common."

Following the youth meeting, my friend and I decided we would each meet someone. I approached Reggie and began to talk to him. I liked the idea that he was both a doctor and a Jew, and I became very interested in him. But I was cautious. At that time it would have been unthinkable for me to marry outside of my religion. I needed to find out more about Reggie and Chiropractic, because it seemed it was the only thing Reggie talked about.

Reggie did have one other passion at this time, and it was playing bridge.* Again, just by coincidence, I'd learned to play bridge just three weeks earlier. That's how the romance began. We talked Chiropractic and went to bridge clubs and played competitive bridge. Bridge clubs were another excellent way to meet people and spread the word about Chiropractic.

When Reggie came to my home to meet my father Max they immediately hit it off. My father had a better relationship with Reggie then he did with any of his own children, and Reggie got along with my father better than he did his own. Although my father wasn't educated, he had a great mind, and he respected Reggie because he was educated, and so well read. It also helped that Reggie wasn't a snob of any kind, he just loved people.

* Contract bridge, usually known simply as bridge, is a trick-taking card game played by four players in two competing partnerships.

Reggie loved to discuss and get completely engrossed in subjects. He could talk and listen for hours. He and dad would lock themselves into a corner of the house and play chess and discuss politics for hours. It wasn't fluff; they deeply discussed world politics and the effects it had on civilization.

Our relationship progressed, but we were both broke, so we continued playing bridge and going to Chiropractic meetings. At that time I was far more interested in Reggie than in Chiropractic. During this time I suffered from terrible migraine headaches. One time Reggie saw me taking an aspirin and it really upset him. He told me he didn't want to date someone who took drugs, so I took my last pill in December, 1958.

What really sold me on Reggie and Chiropractic was seeing him take care of his mother. That Reggie could be so loving and completely caring sold me on him. In those days, you didn't see *any* men act like he did. He had a tenderness about him that was like a mother bird tending a nest. Reggie was so passionate about people and Chiropractic that it touched my heart.

His mother's seven strokes, coupled with her heavy British accent, made it hard for me to understand her. She had bilateral pitting edema that caused her legs to swell out terribly.

When she first arrived, we took her to the shoe store to try to find her shoes, but we could only get some oversized slippers. Reggie adjusted her side posture (atlas only) and one week later the edema was gone! I was so impressed that you could adjust the atlas on a 60 year old and the body changed as a result. You have to understand that as a public health nurse, I thought I'd seen it all, but here was something I'd never even dreamed about! I couldn't believe it. Chiropractic was like a miracle to me.

Reggie's mother lived with his sister, who worked full-time, and wasn't able to take her to the Chiropractor as often as needed. It was decided that the best place for Reggie's mother was with Reggie, so she moved into the office with him. She slept in the resting booth at the back of the office.

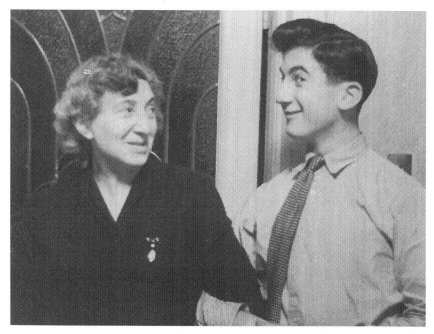

Reggie was devoted to his mother. He was the most caring man I have ever met.

-Irene Gold

At that time, people with pitting edema were put on low salt diets and loads of drugs, and we rarely saw much change at all. This woman changed nothing in her diet; in fact, she loved Chinese food and ate it all the time. She did everything opposite of what we'd been taught in nursing school and got incredible results. My mind was racing with the practical results that Chiropractic care could bring to the public.

I decided it was time to make a good impression on Reggie, so I invited him over for dinner. In my family I was considered quite a cook. I prepared my best meal, which was boiled chicken and boiled vegetables. As I later learned, it was a pretty tasteless, totally forgettable meal. The next week Reggie offered to come over and cook a meal for my entire family. He cooked incredible lasagna which was full of flavor. My family had never even cooked with salt! Reggie showed us the way, and we learned what food should taste like! That's how Reggie was to me, he brought full flavor and light into my life.

I was terribly shy, not even able to get up in front of a crowd and say my name. I viewed myself as a plain person. Because of my upbringing, I had no confidence whatsoever. I thought that males were important, but not females. Reggie changed all that. We began to cook together and make meals together in my kitchen. The times Reggie and I sat in my kitchen talking and cooking are some of the most pleasant memories I have. It was a magical time in my life.

I was still taking classes at Columbia University when Reggie and I began dating. Reggie used to come by and help me with my homework. It was a way for us to spend time together. Sometimes I had a class in literature or history and I would have to read books and then write papers. One time I had to write a paper on Hemmingway. I read the book and explained it to Reggie in detail.

However, I was still having a tough time writing my paper. I just couldn't write a sensible report. I told Reggie my problem, and he then proceeded to dictate the entire report. I wrote it down word for word, it was unbelievable! We didn't have to go back even one time or change a single word.

Chapter 8

Things heat up!

Reggie and I had been dating for about nine months when I decided this dating stuff would have to end. It was either marriage or nothing. When I first met Reggie I couldn't believe anyone like him would be interested in me. Even though I was flattered by all the attention Reggie gave me, my sensible upbringing taught me to always rely on myself. Reggie was about ten years older than me and really didn't want to get married.

Reggie had a fairly serious relationship with a woman while he was in Palmer, and after he and I had been dating a while this girl called him. She wanted to meet with Reggie to discuss getting back together again. When Reggie told me, my heart dropped. A second later I came back to my senses. I never told Reggie what he should do. He stammered and went on about how I was the girl for him, but he just wanted to meet with this other girl to talk it all out. I was having none of it!

Reggie went to meet her, so I made myself unavailable. I went to a friend's house one town over and told absolutely no one where I was. I left on a Friday and came back late on Sunday night. When I got home, my sister told me Reggie had been calling for two days straight, and every ten minutes on Sunday. That was it! I knew I had him, or at least got his attention.

Reggie still really did not want to get married. I told him that he had a choice to make. I couldn't go on being his girlfriend forever. I wanted more out of life than that. So I went down to the Navy recruitment center and obtained the papers to become a Navy nurse. There was a three year enlistment. After serving three years, the Navy would pay for any education I would want. They were also going to let me sign up as an officer because of my training in nursing. I showed Reggie the papers, and told him to make a decision. If you don't want me, fine, but you'll never see me again. I told him I was enlisting in three months, so he had to make a decision.

Reggie knew I wasn't kidding, and I wasn't. Within a couple of days he came around and said I was right, let's do this thing. It was the right time for us. He was working hard trying to get his practice started, and I knew everybody in town. I also helped him in the office.

Marriages are a partnership, and we had lots of things in common. We both wanted to help people and we both always did everything full tilt. Neither of us ever did anything just to get by. We did everything to the best of our ability. We knew that you had to get better at whatever you were doing if you just kept doing your best.

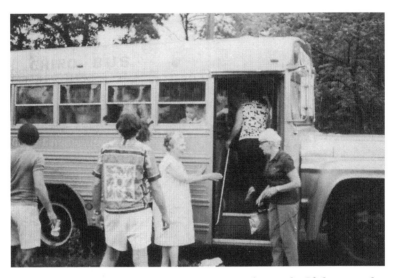

There was no excuse for not getting adjusted. If the people couldn't get to us, we'd come to them with the "Gold Bus." We had bus stops posted around town.

Chapter 9

Building the office in Spring Valley

"All great thinkers get information from somewhere. Some get it through the outside in educated ways, and others get it through direct innate to innate contact."

-Judd Nogrady

Judd

When I was approached about writing this book with Irene, my first thought was that they have the wrong man. I had absolutely no knowledge of Reggie, I never heard him speak, nor had I ever read anything he'd written. In fact, I wasn't even sure who he was other than Irene's husband. It was my opinion he had *absolutely nothing* to do with me or the way I practiced Chiropractic. However, as I interviewed people for this book I was amazed to find that I was completely wrong! In fact, Reggie was responsible for my improved health and my family evolution into principled Chiropractic.

When Reggie was in practice he used the famous "Gold Bus" to help patients get to the office. The "Gold Bus" ran three days per week. The bus had an incredible young Chiropractor named Dr. Jay Kauffman at the wheel. Dr. Jay learned straight Chiropractic from Reggie, who turned on another young, eager, but lost Chiropractor named Dr. Adam Nogrady, who is my brother.

When my brother graduated from Logan College in 1988, he was completely confused. He'd received a great medical education. Logan had not only taught medical Chiropractic, but the college had lectured strongly that "straight Chiropractic was ruining Chiropractic."

The organization at Logan put such an emphasis on the negativity of "straight Chiropractic" that Adam viewed it as a disease.

When he graduated, it was customary to go to the "mixer" store and pick out your machines and the various modalities that were all "necessary" to begin practice. At the mixer store they put together a package price for you, and then when you found your location, they shipped it to you.

My brother, true to his education, went to the "mixer" store and put together his order, but he hesitated on sealing the deal with payment because he really didn't know where he wanted to practice. Besides, something just seemed wrong to him. The more he looked at all those machines the more he got this inner feeling something was wrong. He wanted to help people, but his education didn't allow him to be a medical doctor, and it didn't allow him to be a real Chiropractor. He just didn't have the tools.

My brother was looking for offices all over New York State. This was well before the internet, so in those days looking meant driving all over. In one particular town there is a bridge that separates New York from Pennsylvania. As my brother approached the bridge, he decided to take a look around in Pennsylvania. This made no sense because he wasn't licensed in Pennsylvania, and he didn't know anyone there. But he had this inner feeling that he just had to cross that bridge.

As soon as he crossed the bridge he came into a small town that looked just like all the small towns on the New

York side. He was about to turn around and go back when he saw a sign, "Dr. Jay Kauffman – Straight Chiropractic." It was the word "straight" that really caught my brother's attention. Here was one of the witch doctors that Logan College had warned him about. It was a Sunday morning so my brother was sure the office would be closed, but he just had to look in and lay his eyes on the enemy's lair. He quietly wheeled into the parking lot. Before he could get out and take a quick peek, another car pulled up and the person got out and walked in.

My brother decided to go into the forbidden zone. As he stepped through the door his fears were fully realized. He'd been taught that every respectable doctor wore a suit, tie, and white jacket, but here was Dr. Jay, adjusting the entire high school football team while wearing Bermuda shorts and a Hawaiian print short sleeve shirt. No one can quite wear this ensemble like Dr. Jay. Jay had a way about him that really made the bright red Hawaiian shirt and deep blue Bermuda pants stand out with his bright white sneakers.

My brother's first reaction was that all the instructors at Logan were right, these straight practitioners really were the devil, and here was living proof! This was my brother's first time seeing people get checked. As he watched Dr. Jay checking people, his attitude changed. He saw player after player get off the table happy, thankful and exuberant about the Chiropractic adjustment they'd just received. My brother's life changed. He now realized he needed to understand what this was all about.

As Jay checked the last player, he turned to my brother and introduced himself. My brother couldn't contain himself. He began asking questions immediately, but Dr. Jay held up one gigantic paw like hand and said, "Stop. Where are you staying now?"

Adam explained that he was living with our grandparents.

"Call them and tell them you will be home very late, and then we'll start discussing straight Chiropractic."

After Jay finished, which took them through lunch, dinner, and lots of time in between, my brother was converted to straight Chiropractic.

A short time later, Adam was still looking for a practice location when he "accidently" met a kindly gentleman named Paul Proulx while purchasing gasoline. As my brother talked and asked his new found friend Paul about buildings for rent, Paul asked him what kind of work he was in. My brother answered, "Chiropractic."

Paul asked, "What kind of Chiropractor are you?"

"Straight" my brother answered.

A broad grin spread across Paul's face. "In that case, I have a place for you."

Dr. Paul was a straight Chiropractor. Paul was an early Palmer graduate and also a friend of Jay. Within days my brother was in practice with two mentors, Dr. Jay Kaufman and Dr. Paul Proulx.

Dr. Paul gave my brother the first month's rent free, and sent him many new patients to help him get his new practice going. (The conversion of my brother by Jay led me to get adjusted by Paul, whose upper cervical toggle recoil adjustment changed my life).

My brother's practice took off to over 750 patients per week within two years, and stayed at that level for 15 years. When I went to Chiropractic college years later, I encouraged fellow students to come home with me on breaks and see how Chiropractic should be practiced. The one student that came home with me and took to heart what he saw was Liam Schübel. 25 years later Liam introduced me to Irene, for the purpose of writing this book. Without ever knowing it until now, Reggie has been a huge influence on my life in Chiropractic.

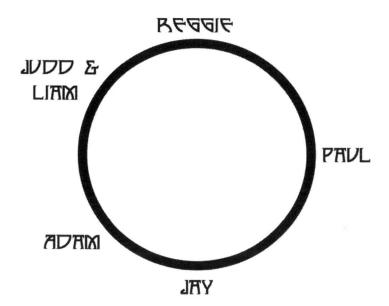

Chapter 10

The practice years

Reggie's office opened in 1958. First, some construction was needed inside in order to accommodate a Chiropractic office. The construction workers were some of Reggie's first patients. They were a captive audience, and Reggie reminded them that if they wanted to get paid, they had to tell others about Chiropractic.

The office was located on the main street in Spring Valley. Reggie was a people person, and every morning he went out and introduced himself at businesses throughout town. He went to the same place for coffee and he quickly became a regular. In this fashion he met many of the same people, and he always talked Chiropractic. There'd been many Chiropractors in Spring Valley, and all of them lasted about six months, and then moved on. Spring Valley was not a Chiropractic-friendly town, as there was a strong medical presence, and they protected their turf. At this time there was no licensure, no insurance and no advertising allowed. In fact, if you advertised, you got investigated and brought up on charges for practicing medicine without a license.

Reggie was absolutely fascinated with Chiropractic. Everything we did revolved around it. One of the first things we did was start meeting other Chiropractors, and when we met, we all talked Chiropractic.

One of the first people Reggie fellowshipped with was Bill Bahan from Derry, New Hampshire. The Bahan's were a huge Chiropractic family. There were ten children in total. Five became Chiropractors and the other five married Chiropractors. The Bahan family would have meetings and about 50 Chiropractors would show up. We'd talk about Chiropractic principles, and discuss the best way to introduce Chiropractic to lay people. We could talk Chiropractic all night! We felt drawn together by a common mission: we wanted to represent Chiropractic to the world, and we were committed to bringing the best we had to offer.

Reggie was speaking to different groups of lay people throughout New York State. They helped him pick up a patient here and there, but just as often they provided new patients for the Chiropractor in the town he was visiting. He also gave talks to groups of his patients' friends. Reggie would travel almost anywhere as long as he could spread the Chiropractic message.

We were making a living in Chiropractic, but not much more than that. I was working at my job and Reggie was just getting by. In November, 1960, Dr. Napolitano, the President of Columbia Institute of Chiropractic, asked Reggie if he would teach philosophy at the school. Initially, he asked Reggie to come in one day per week. At that time Columbia had day and evening classes, so Reggie would drive about an hour into New York City, teach the morning class, then hang around through the middle of the day and teach the class at night. This one day per week, part-time thing wound up being a four and half year commitment. It also became a three full days per week commitment when the school dropped the evening classes.

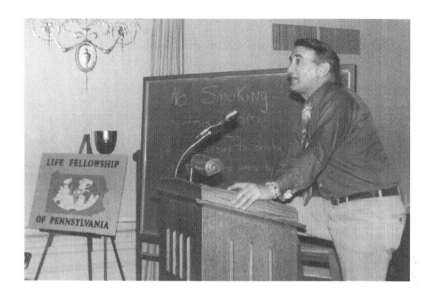

Reggie always insisted on $1 per year as his annual salary. He felt that teaching philosophy and teaching others how to discuss Chiropractic was his duty. Many people don't understand the depth of commitment Reggie had for Chiropractic and other Chiropractors. He felt that it was far more important to live a fruitful life than to chase dollars. He believed that education should enable us to better serve our fellow man. No one has the right to travel the road of life without paying his passage, and Reggie made sure that he paid his way.

Dr. Napolitano hated to travel, so he sent Reggie to state conventions, and Reggie became quite well known as a speaker. When he finally stopped representing the school, he had over 150 state plaques. Reggie spoke in every state, multiple times. After his speeches he often got requests from organizations within the state to speak at different group functions.

All this speaking was great for Reggie, because it gave him a way to voice his new ideas about Chiropractic. However, it didn't help us financially. We still lived in the office with our hot plate, foldaway couch and little else. This simple little place was our home for four and a half years. Being a bit more practical, I finally told Reggie we should move. It's one thing having a home office but quite another having an office as your home. The subject of moving was upsetting to Reggie. He didn't want to spend extra money on what he considered to be unnecessary things, and he thought anything above our meager surroundings was unnecessary.

In rare instances, Reggie's temper flashed. He couldn't understand why I wanted to spend "all this money" when "we had everything." I knew him well enough to let the matter drop. I knew he had his own way of working things out in his mind. He needed to turn problems over in his mind and consider all sides. He would take his time, thinking of all possible ideas. Three tense days later, Reggie asked me to go out with him for a drive.

He took me to see a bi-level three bedroom home with four columns on the outside, and asked me if I thought it would make me happy. I asked him, "Why are you showing me a house when we have a perfectly good living space? You said so yourself."

"I've been thinking of having a house just like this built on the land your father gave us for our wedding present," he said. That's how Reggie was. He could see it was reasonable to move, but it still had to be his idea. We moved into the house on 2 Ellish Parkway in December, 1964.

In April, 1965, he got fired from his $1 dollar a year job. The school wanted to go in a different direction, and one of the things they felt they needed to do to get ahead was to join the American Chiropractic Association (ACA). More and more schools were being lured away from traditional Chiropractic, and the ACA promised more lucrative times ahead. In order to join the ACA, the school felt they had to change their philosophy. In order to do this, Napolitano knew he couldn't keep Reggie around. So the ACA was in and Reggie and his philosophy were out. April 1 was Reggie's last day.

Reggie had the ability to move on quickly. It wasn't that he wasn't emotionally hurt by the treatment he received from people, but he just knew that feeling sorry for himself wasn't productive. When people threw him a real big curve or outright denounced him, he quickly rebounded by caring for Chiropractic more than his own personal feelings. In Chiropractic, he saw something larger and more important than himself.

On April 30, he held a large lay lecture for his regular patients and told them all to bring friends. We rented a large hall. Reggie could finally put his full effort and abilities into running his practice. He gave it everything he had, and the people responded en masse. Over the next month we started over 250 new families, not individuals, but families. From the beginning, we always spoke of the importance of the entire family being under care. It was an anomaly that a person started alone unless he had no family.

Reggie also became one of the first sports Chiropractors. An early patient was Floyd Patterson, a famous world champion boxer. His manager felt Floyd was too valuable to risk trying Chiropractic, so he sent the sparing partners to Reggie to get adjusted first. The sparing partners had such dramatic increases in their abilities that Floyd felt he had to get adjusted also. Floyd got no special treatment from Reggie, but had to go through patient education and pay just like everyone else.

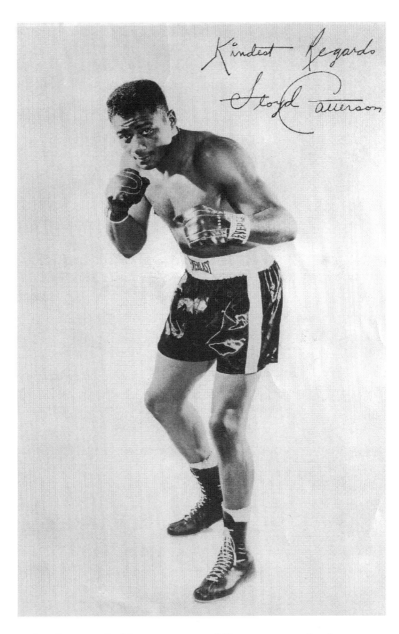

Dr. Reggie Gold accompanied Patterson to the Ingemar Johansson fight, both Sonny Liston fights, and his battle with Mohammed Ali in 1965.

At that time we had a box on the wall, and people were encouraged to pay whatever they could afford based on their income and life situation. By having a box we felt that people would never feel like they couldn't come and receive care.

Floyd never handled his own money; everything was done through his attorney. Floyd decided he could afford seventy dollars per visit and had his accountant send a check each time he was checked. As Floyd began to see and understand the benefits Chiropractic care gave him, he asked if Reggie would travel to his training camp in Florida for six weeks. Reggie loved to travel, and jumped at the chance to promote Chiropractic.

This was the early 1960's. The southern part of the United States was still segregated. It was shocking to Reggie, coming from New York, to find that Floyd couldn't stay in the same hotel with him because of segregation. That a world champion boxer couldn't stay in the same hotel was unbelievable to him.

Floyd also wanted Reggie in his corner during the fight in case he needed to be checked or adjusted. When Floyd won the title he gave credit to Chiropractic, and a large article in Sports Illustrated talked about it.

Reggie was the New York State representative to the ICA and later became even more involved. I was in the women's organization that raised money to put Chiropractic books in public libraries, and that raised money for Chiropractic scholarships. One of the contributions that I made was a hooked rug that said "Chiropractic keeps me smiling." That rug took me an entire year to finish, and it was a labor of love. We raffled it off for the youth organization.

Youth and student groups are so very important. Many of these kids, who were about 15 or 16 years old when they joined the youth group, went on to become Chiropractors. So many young people got a good start in life from our youth group organization.

I was an active Chiropractic wife. I still had my own career, but I fully supported Reggie and Chiropractic. When Reggie left the Columbian Institute of Chiropractic, he started having meetings at our house. These were all organized by telephone.

By this time, the Bahan family had drifted out of Chiropractic philosophy and begun a spiritualist movement. Bill Bahan believed that if you lived a life in complete contact with the innate you would never die. Reggie couldn't take this wishful thinking seriously, and he denounced it as an idea that did not fit within any of the principles of Chiropractic.

Bill Bahan moved to Loveland, Colorado with many of his followers to a large commune, where they followed the beliefs of Ontology, which is more like a spiritualist religion, separate from the ideas and principles of Chiropractic. When Bill Bahan was in Chiropractic, he practiced with his four brothers. They had two offices, three doctors in one and two in the other. They saw over 1,000 people on any given Friday. The offices had 150 chairs in each waiting room.

As they drifted away from straight Chiropractic, they began to adjust without contact and instead did adjustments through the air in side posture position. They began to see themselves as pure spiritualist healers. Bill Bahan was so charismatic that he could pull anybody in with just his smile. He had an incredible impact on people. He spoke from the heart. He was not political, he was authentic, and he was a 100% honest, pure, and kind person. But he had philosophical differences that were far from straight Chiropractic.

Many of the Chiropractors that were regulars at the early home meetings came to every meeting. At that time, colleges were instilling fear of straight Chiropractic, and students were strongly warned about attending Chiropractic meetings. We decided on nine house meetings per year. We always had at least 50 people, and some of our larger meetings were attended by over 200. It was amazing that we all packed into a ranch home basement!

The office on 2 Ellish Parkway was on a corner lot with beautiful landscaping. I can still see the spring flowers. We had a small waiting room with 15 chairs, and as we got busy people would wait outside. We were open seven days per week, and on Sunday mornings the police would come and direct traffic. We got so busy that we graduated to the number system, "bakery style." People took a number and then went to church, came back and got checked.

We didn't design the house layout ourselves. It was a complete copy of the house that Reggie had originally showed me. The only exception was we converted the two car garage into our office. Now we lived in a house with an office rather than an office that doubled as a house. The two car garage was divided into three rooms, a waiting room, and two adjusting rooms, one large and one small.

In the smaller room we had a Pucket table which mounted against the wall. The patient would sit on a chair and a toggle recoil adjustment was made with the patient in the seated position. The big room had a Hi-lo and side posture table.

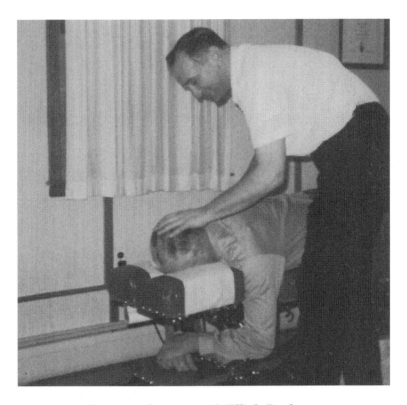

Reggie adjusting at 2 Ellish Parkway

Within one month of getting "fired" things really took off at the office. Reggie was 100% committed. He gave up all outside things and dedicated his complete focus to seeing people and speaking from the heart. We went from 60 patients per day to 100 per day, and then within the year, we had 240 people on a Sunday morning. This forced us to be open seven days a week, and we hired associates. This was a completely different practice then he'd had for the last six years. The house meetings were necessary for Reggie. He had to share Chiropractic, because talking Chiropractic philosophy was as natural to him as breathing.

Evening Sun, Hanover, PA - August 23, 1972

When the word got out about how good Reggie was at bringing in new patients, he was asked to do layman's lectures for other Chiropractors in their home towns. Reggie did layman lectures for Chiropractors in the field about 40 weeks per year. He went to Jim Sigafoose's chicken dinner and was asked to do the layman's lecture. It was a big honor for Reggie because he loved to communicate the message.

At this time I was still working as a nurse, and referring people to Chiropractic whenever possible. Nursing was very satisfying to me. Chiropractic was just more advanced than medicine. Getting the body to function optimally was and is a whole lot smarter than treating disease.

I started getting ideas that I should advance myself and become a Chiropractor. There were two instances that made the decision for me. In 1971, we'd just finished a large house meeting and picked a date for the next one. After everybody left, Reggie realized that he'd be in Hawaii doing a lecture, so he asked me to do it for him. I fought this. I was too nervous, and I didn't think I could speak well enough to give real value to a large group of Chiropractors, many of whom would have traveled large distances to attend.

We gave two patient lectures in the office, one that was open to a group, and one in private. In the beginning Reggie did both, but as we got busy, I did the private lectures and he did the group. While I was experienced giving the private lectures for new patients, I was terrified at the thought of speaking at the house meeting, so Reggie got two Chiropractors to cover for me. When the first guy dropped out I wasn't too worried, but when the second guy, Mario, called and said that his daughter got hurt and he couldn't make it, I was beside myself!

The morning of the lecture I was a bit relieved, because it was snowing, and I figured no one would show up! But by four o'clock it had cleared up, and over a hundred people came. I put on a brave face and gave my layman's lecture. I did my best. As a result, I got numerous letters and calls of congratulations. I'll never forget the one from Dr. Ron Peek. He wrote to say it was the best understanding he'd ever had of how to relate Chiropractic to a patient. These letters and calls really boosted my confidence. For the first time I really felt as if I could do it.

A month later I went to my first and last Dynamic Essentials. DE was a seminar that was put on by Dr. Sid Williams, the founder of Life College. Reggie was a regular speaker at DE every three months, for four years. When the speakers were finished they had an open mike, and people could get up and say a few words about how they felt. Linda Elwart, an 18 year old from Michigan, got up and said there was no question in her mind here and now, she was going to commit her life to Chiropractic. I sat there stunned! I was thinking "I am twice her age, I have been living my life in Chiropractic all these years, why don't I do it?"

I didn't think I could be a doctor, but then I realized if others could do it, so could I. Unfortunately, it was the last DE that Reggie ever spoke at. This was because he was so disheartened at the sale of medical equipment at a Chiropractic seminar, as well as the promotion of concept therapy, that he verbally denounced both from the stage, which earned him a lifetime ban.

Chapter 11

The truth must prevail

At my nursing job I was a school nurse, but this position was going to be changed, so I was offered an administrative position. As a school nurse, I had to give medical advice, but I knew it was wrong advice. I wasn't allowed to discuss Chiropractic with people, and this really bothered me. I had to give Chiropractic advice "under the table" as it were, and that's not who I am. I like to be very straightforward and direct. It was one thing to have to sneak Chiropractic in as a nurse. As an administrator, I would be expected to write the rules, and I just couldn't do this if it excluded Chiropractic. There was no way they were going to let straight Chiropractic be discussed.

I had to do an interview with a woman whose daughter was doing poorly in school. I went in to interview her and learned that she'd been in an auto accident. Since the accident she'd been having convulsions. I began to give her a Chiropractic lecture, and while doing so, she had a grand mal seizure. There was a piece of a doll on the floor, I think it was a doll's arm, so I quickly shoved the dolls arm into her mouth to keep her teeth open. As she came out of the seizure she was thankful, because it was the first time she didn't bite her tongue. I finished the talk and shortly afterward she started Chiropractic care and started to get better.

I thought of this for a long time. How could I be part of a medical system that denied people the chance to get better? It really ate at me. I knew deep down inside I had to become a Chiropractor.

I decided to go to the Columbia Institute of Chiropractic, now called New York Chiropractic College, because it was less than an hour from my house, and it gave me the opportunity to stay involved with the office while I went to school. The office was doing very well, so we figured it was a great time for me to start Chiropractic college.

We hired a Chiropractor to work in the office full-time as an associate. He was a graduate of the now defunct New York Institute, who had failed in practice and was working in a shoe store. Now the office was covered seven days a week. We thought the world of him – until our great associate decided he was going to go out on his own and take our patients with him.

In the meantime, the local Chiropractors were upset with Reggie because he was doing so well. We had a Chiropractic bus, which was painted solid gold, and it was driven by Jay Kauffman, who had just graduated. Jay would pick people up, bring them to the office to get adjusted, and then drive them home. We even posted our own bus stops!

After the first associate left we hired another, and the troubles kept coming. Some of the local Chiropractors turned us in for a completely bogus charge. I have to admit, it was an ingenious way to get back at us, and it cast a deep suspicion on us. Reggie was turned in for practicing under an assumed name. This was big news, and it hit the front page of the local newspapers, claiming that somehow we were not really who we said we were. (I've never figured out who they were claiming we were supposed to be).

They timed the charge perfectly, as Reggie was out of the country, in South Africa, giving a lecture. This gave a whole lot of time for "the charge" to become known in the community, and there was no way for him to answer it.

The front page of our local paper was sensational. They acted like they'd captured a foreign spy or some such nonsense. It was all just a well-organized smear campaign. They never said what his real name was supposed to be, they just emphasized that he was a fraud. The name they referred to was "Gold Chiropractic Office." The paper called me and I told them "Gold" was our name, period, and there was nothing to discuss. I was astounded that it was legal to make up stories such as this.

I was served with papers and informed that when Reggie got home he had had to appear before the board. Of course with all of this negative publicity most of the patients stopped coming in, and the associate was not in a position to straighten things out. This really devastated the office. The other associate left and took whatever patients he could.

I really loved the practicality of Chiropractic, but I was shocked by the politics and the mean-spirited vindictiveness of the board.

When Reggie came back the office was almost at a standstill. He answered the charges which were, of course, totally bogus. If they had done an ounce of investigation before they went on their witch hunt, they would have known it was all nonsense. However, they didn't care what the truth was, they just wanted to damage our reputation. Finally, about six weeks later, an apology was printed on page 11, hidden from view. It took six months of hard work before we got everything straightened out.

With our new associate things began to look up, but then he wasn't as honest as he could have been, and we had to let him go. It was as if we were starting from scratch. When things started going well again, the board charged us with advertising, which was illegal in New York State, because the bus had our name on it.

Reggie again answered the charges and then started to build again. He had the attitude that once things were done you moved on and never looked back. With a lot of hard work the office started to grow again.

With thoughts of enlightening the world and helping the Chiropractic profession, as well as individual Chiropractors, Reggie began to revitalize Patients Association for Chiropractic Education (PACE). Reggie wanted the public to become informed about Chiropractic. It was his idea that once the public really knew what Chiropractic care was capable of, people would start to utilize Chiropractic care, and this would help all Chiropractors. He felt that when people began to get and stay adjusted, Chiropractic could lift humanity. He had a vision of Chiropractic leading the world's people to a higher level of existence.

PACE was first started in the 1930's by Dr. Bill Werner, a Chiropractor from Queens, New York. Dr. Bill was filled with love for humanity and a deep love for Chiropractic. This compassion and commitment poured out of him. He filled Madison Square Garden with 15,000 people for a layman's lecture in 1932. PACE was an organization of Chiropractic patients that advocated the benefits of Chiropractic.

Bill died in 1957. He had two children, both of whom went to Chiropractic college. Bill's widow was a good friend of ours, and she told us many stories about him and Chiropractic.

Bill also faced many difficulties because he was so popular. Out of jealousy, some Chiropractors made phony complaints against him, and tried to make his life miserable in general. When his widow explained it all to us, it made us realize that when you stick your neck out, there's always someone trying to chop it off.

The whole idea of PACE really resonated with Reggie. We had a very active patient who became the president of PACE. We offered chapters to other Chiropractors, and once per year we met with all PACE chapters. The patients were really tight, and they understood Chiropractic.

PACE was started the same year that the rubella vaccine got started. We found out that the medics were putting on a radio show promoting the rubella vaccine. We had a patient that was permanently damaged from this vaccine, so we got one of our patients to go to one of the medical society meetings posing as a journalist. He found out what they were planning to do and when they were going to do it, so we knew exactly what they were going to say, and when.

The PACE organization bought and paid for advertising time on the same radio station as the medical society's radio show. On the show they'd talk about how great the vaccine was and that everybody should get it, and then went to the commercial. Then the commercial would say "my daughter took the rubella vaccine and she has permanent damage," and explain what was wrong with her. Every time they took a break, we had an anti-rubella vaccination ad. This was all done through PACE.

While people have to be told about Chiropractic, they also need to be informed about the dangers of drugs. The world is literally dying from prescription and over the counter medications. Although Chiropractic is not about drug or medic bashing, someone needs to tell the truth about drugs and the devastating effects they are having on our country and the planet.

We also had a mall program where patients would hand out balloons that said "keep smiling", and patients would go out and talk to people. We'd invite Chiropractors to come do postural analysis in booths that were setup.

Chiropractic students were invited to join in to explain the benefits and the philosophy of Chiropractic. We were not concerned with only getting Reggie new clients; we wanted all people to know about the benefits of Chiropractic so they could seek care wherever they lived. I will never forget our biggest mall event, it was advertised all over, and we got a tremendous turnout. Unfortunately, not one of my classmates showed up to help. They missed an opportunity of a lifetime!

I started at 10am and finished at 10pm. I personally spoke to over 700 people that day, sometimes one on one and other times in small groups. We found Chiropractors for them in their hometowns. We did this on a Saturday and signed up 35 new patients for Reggie's office, and signed up over 100 people for other Chiropractors in the area.

When people rejected me, I never got upset, I just moved on the next person. My attitude was, "I am here to help you and educate you on having a better life! If you don't want an education and a better life, then get lost!" The public had been brainwashed into becoming pill addicts. It was very difficult for them to accept a new idea, but I always felt so terrible that their children wouldn't get the chance at a better life. Failure to reach people motivated me to get better at communicating the message. Then I'd find some who did want to hear the message, and I gave them my best. By the end of the day I was tired, but thankful for the chance to promote Chiropractic.

PACE was all about getting the public educated about Chiropractic. We'd run lecture a once a year for all the patients and invite them to bring someone along. There was a dinner after the meeting. At one of these meetings we had 500 people. It would've been more, but the hall we rented could only hold that many. We turned away more than 600 people! As we spread the word about Chiropractic, our office grew to 800 then to over 1,000 visits per week.

As we got more experienced with politics we tried to do things a little smarter. We'd always hold the meeting at a time when a local politician wanted an audience. There were always elections in November, so we held our meeting in October, and invited them to come in for ten minutes. Sometimes the politicians would learn a little about Chiropractic. We always hoped they would help spread the word.

One of the main concerns Reggie and I had was patient retention. Starting people was one thing, but making sure they understood lifetime care was another. It was very important to us. It was great that they got the message, but were they telling their neighbors and friends? And were they having their children checked? Helping children have healthy lives and healthy spines is so important. We knew that in order for people to accept a new idea, a onetime Chiropractic explanation wasn't enough. We knew a continuing education program was vitally important.

Chapter 12

Going Where?

The office was back to running fairly well. I was working in the office and going to Columbia. I remember thinking "finally things are running smoothly" when Thom Gelardi called.

Thom was unhappy with what was happening at Palmer. It was Thom's opinion that pure Chiropractic was not going to survive unless we did something. He wanted to start a school so straight Chiropractic would survive, and that upper cervical technique would be taught. Thom made all the arrangements with Michael Kale. Thom put it together, Michael was going to be the Vice President and Thom was going to be the President. At this time Reggie and I thought it was a great idea and agreed to help.

As we started to gather students for the new school, Reggie and I joked that you could call yourself whatever you wanted, but without students it wasn't much of a school. We made getting students a top priority.

Thom and Reggie knew each other from their Palmer days. Later, Thom was the ICA representative from South Carolina and Reggie was the representative from New York. Every time the ICA wanted to change anything or do something to undermine straight Chiropractic, Reggie and Thom were always on the same side.

It seemed that the ICA was always trying to adopt something more or include something else into Chiropractic. Thom and Reggie felt that Chiropractic was near perfect in its pure form. They both felt that adding anything to Chiropractic only diluted and weakened it.

The ICA loved to use the words "preparatory to and complementary of", and then tried to include every procedure under the sun. Reggie and Thom wanted to keep it straight. They could see physical therapy (PT) coming in and they knew that PT was just the tip of the iceberg.

As Thom explained his vision for Sherman, Reggie could see the need of a place to keep it pure. Thom knew that Reggie had contacts in all 50 states and several countries. He also knew Reggie could motivate a group of people to take action. Most of all Thom knew that once Reggie put his mind to something, he worked on it with all of his substantial energy. Thom was astute enough to understand that Reggie was a huge asset at getting people behind the school.

Thom and Michael came from South Carolina to visit us in New York to discuss the school, and we all went to dinner together. We decided to go to a nearby Italian restaurant. The restaurant didn't have a liquor license, so it was customary to bring your own alcohol. Reggie and I enjoyed good wine with our meal, so I packed two large bottles of wine. The restaurant was a ten minute car ride from our house. I told Reggie I would drive so he could talk with the guys. If I'd known what was going to happen I would have made Reggie drive!

Thom was doing all the talking and Reggie was doing all the listening. After about a minute of conversation, Thom says "Reggie, I want you to work at the school full time!" Nine minutes later when we got to the restaurant

Reggie had agreed to move to South Carolina! I was in complete shock!

During the meal they discussed when and how the school would run and what they'd do. They had complete confidence that the school would open and succeed. I sat there stunned. I decided it was a good idea to have a drink, so I opened the two bottles of wine and then found out that Michael and Thom don't drink, so Reggie and I finished both bottles, and then I drove home. I am not sure if I was drunk or in shock, but I was absolutely flabbergasted.

It was the spring of 1973, and I was still in Chiropractic college. When I wasn't in class or clinic, Reggie and I were recruiting in Spring Valley and throughout New York and New Jersey. We had lots of help once the word of what we were doing got out. Many straight Chiropractors from all over gave their support in many ways. Getting Sherman started was a real group effort.

There was one sour note before the school officially opened: Michael and Thom had a falling out. It was decided that Reggie would start as Dean. Reggie wanted to practice in South Carolina, because our plan was that we were going to open an office and run the school simultaneously. Reggie took the test to get a license, which was given in an informal way. Everyone was in one large room, and they were all talking to each other in between stations while in the testing room.

The exam was basic and straightforward. So much so that Reggie fully expected to pass easily. But before they would even grade Reggie's test, the South Carolina Board dropped a bombshell and accused Reggie of cheating! This effectively denied him a license and ruined any chance of him opening a practice in a timely fashion. Reggie had no alternative but to file a lawsuit against the South Carolina Board. The whole fiasco really took a toll on him; it was difficult to focus on the school and his lawsuit at the same time.

The battle for his right to licensure brought a lot of political grief to the school. Later, the South Carolina Chiropractic Board brought pressure on the school to dismiss Reggie. The threat was that if the school didn't get rid of Reggie, it would not get accreditation.

The South Carolina Board began using any tricks they could to keep new graduates from gaining licensure. I took the South Carolina board and failed! Thirty others took the test with me, and only Dr. Myron Brown passed, and he was someone I tutored! I will never forget how ridiculous one part of the exam was. There was an x-ray of the knee. It looked all messed up and diseased to me, but it turned out it was Michael Kale's normal knee! We hadn't studied extremities on x-ray when I was in school because the law did not allow anyone to x-ray below the second lumbar vertebra.

When Joe Felcia's wife Katie graduated and took the South Carolina board, they interviewed her. At that time there were two women and two men on the board. The members of the board couldn't handle the idea that she was going to practice on her own. It was 1974, and they said a woman couldn't practice on her own! In the interview they asked her who she was going to work for. When she said she would be working on her own, they asked her, "What does your mother think about a young women working without a male in the office?" She was speechless. What made it even more galling was that there were two women on the board in collusion with this type of nonsense!

I took the test a second time and failed. During one exam I came close to walking out when I realized that they were using an x-ray physics exam taken from D.D.

Palmer's 1910 text. I finally passed the third exam with a score of 98.

When Reggie began at Sherman, I still had one year left at Columbia. We decided to sell the house, and I moved in with a friend of mine and lived with her for one year until I graduated. That one year was difficult for Reggie and me. Being apart was lonely. We had a great relationship and really valued each other's company, and being in different locations was uncomfortable. We were both willing to bear it for Chiropractic, and we felt it necessary for both of us to continue on our paths, but still it was challenging. I was a full time student and working, and Reggie and I only got to see each other when he came home for a few days. I graduated Chiropractic college in 1974, and began teaching at Sherman on October 1.

For me, it was day one. I taught public health and Genisiology. I'd prepare for weeks and then go through all the material in a matter of days! Teaching was a real eye opener for me. In order to keep classes relevant a lot of material had to be covered.

The last year I worked as a registered nurse I made $15,000. When I put in my resignation, my supervisor called me in and asked me if I was sure I wanted to leave. They offered me a better position and slightly more pay to stay. He explained that between lost salary and tuition it was going to cost me $100,000 to go to school. I looked him in the eye and asked, "Do you think I'm doing this for the money? These are peoples' lives!" Many lay people just don't understand the commitment Chiropractors have to our patients and to the principles of Chiropractic. I started at Sherman for $12,000 per year. A year and a half later I was promoted to Academic Dean, and was paid $20,000.

Reggie started with Sherman in 1973. However, his problems with the board were a real distraction to the school's mission, and his presence was standing in the way of accreditation. It was with a heavy heart that Reggie resigned, leaving in March, 1975. He felt it was best for the school if he stepped aside. This was painful for him, but he knew that the school was off to a good start. He couldn't stand the thought that he in some way would be the reason for the school not gaining accreditation. He wanted the students to have the benefits that accreditation afforded.

I was at Sherman from 1974 through 1978. All together we were in South Carolina for five years.

Chapter 13

The IFCO is born

After Reggie left Sherman he resumed doing seminars and speaking. I was worried for him, but it was needless worry, because he took it all in stride. The benefit was that he could devote his full attention to straight Chiropractic. He really rejoiced at being unrestrained from bureaucracy. He was actually relieved that he could focus his full concentration on creating something lasting for straight Chiropractic.

He loved being involved with the school, but he hated to have to compromise on Chiropractic in any way. He sat down and wrote out the constitution for the Federation of Straight Chiropractors and Organizations (FSCO). (In 2011, FSCO changed their name to IFCO, International Federation of Chiropractors and Organizations). It was obvious that we needed a straight organization, an organization that wouldn't change Chiropractic on a whim, or change it to fit a medical/insurance model or government regulations.

During this time the Council on Chiropractic Education (CCE) became the only accrediting agency. At one time the ICA and the ACA each had their own accrediting organizations. The ICA and the ACA were both invited to Washington to present their proposals for Chiropractic accreditation. Supposedly there was some type of a mix up, and the ACA showed up and the ICA did not, so the

ACA proposal was adopted. When we found out that the ACA was going to run the accreditation for all Chiropractors, we knew that straight Chiropractic was in danger of complete destruction.

We were in complete disbelief when Palmer went with it as well as everyone else. Sherman College did not want to be a part of the CCE. Life College should have been Sherman's companion, but Life decided to accept the rules of the ACA-CCE. Their position was that straight Chiropractic could exist within the rules. I don't know why they wouldn't hold the line, but I think they were willing to compromise in order to maintain accreditation and reap the financial windfall that came with it in the name of federal student loans.

Reggie went to Washington along with Sid Williams and many other people. In the end it was Reggie and Sherman against the CCE. This created a longstanding rift between Sherman and Life. After that it became obvious that we needed another accrediting agency for straight Chiropractic, because we knew that the CCE didn't represent the straight point of view.

Since we had to have accreditation to stay alive, we had to apply or close. The states began to change their laws, requiring a CCE or equivalent accreditation in order for a student to receive a license to practice. Shortly afterward we got a visit from the CCE at Sherman. They examined us inside out and all around and then turned us down for accreditation. During this time, Life went through the same process, but did get accredited. I don't want to detract from Sid Williams, because he did a lot for Chiropractic, but in this instance he put the college in front of Chiropractic. It seems he was willing to bend Chiropractic to fit these new regulations, where Reggie could not.

Chapter 14

ADIO

In Pennsylvania, a group of Chiropractors got together and decided to start ADIO (Above, Down, Inside and Out), which was another straight school. We needed two schools to in order to gain separate accreditation. We started a second accrediting agency called Straight Chiropractic Academic Standards Association (SCASA)*, and at the time we thought Sherman and ADIO could be sister schools. The school's name was Reggie's idea. The idea of the school was discussed by a group of people, and it was decided that Reggie would be the president.

The instructors were mostly graduates from Sherman, and in order for the school to be a financial success, they were told they were to work without pay, just like Reggie did at the Columbia Institute of Chiropractic. Reggie thought all people felt like he did, and that giving back to Chiropractic was an honor. He also thought it was vital that Chiropractic instructors must be successful if they were going to teach anything to students. As the school got started and the instructors got into teaching, many found it was difficult to teach and run practices at the same time. Eventually, many felt they should be paid for teaching. This went against everything Reggie believed in.

SCASA did become an accreditation agency but was dissolved in 1995.

Our first class at ADIO started with over 20 students. It was a well located campus in Levittown, Pennsylvania. Being close to New York and New Jersey, it attracted a lot of people from the tri-state area. We thought the school was off to a great start, but unfortunately many of the teachers were meeting in secret about the situation of pay. They decided they would quit en masse, and would do so during the middle of a semester. They felt this would effectively paralyze the school and force Reggie's hand. (Never mind the terrible situation they would create for the students).

When Reggie was asked to run ADIO, they agreed that he would receive a yearly salary of forty thousand dollars. Reggie never took his salary but instead set up an interest bearing account so the school could earn the 16% interest offered at that time. Reggie wanted the school to be able to draw on the interest while the money sat in the account. Reggie had a five year plan which was to donate all five year's salary in one shot. We had it all worked out with our accountant, for tax purposes it was the best way for us to donate money.

These people didn't understand Reggie's commitment to the ideal of Chiropractic. Reggie would not compromise. He felt that he could get fully committed people. But in the end, the desire to get paid to teach won out, and the instructors walked out. Reggie and I were left with only a handful of loyal teachers. We worked night and day to keep the school open, and we kept the education focused on pure Chiropractic. We were confident that we could find Chiropractors that could teach and be able to have successful practices, or find retired Chiropractors that wanted to give back to the profession.

We were not prepared for how ugly the teachers would be. They had a few more tricks up their sleeve. They got the legislative bodies involved. It was somehow determined that the school could not be accredited by the Commonwealth of Pennsylvania without paid teachers. Those that left thought that when we found out about this requirement we'd take them all back.

They were out to destroy Reggie and me. First they started rumors about me having a lesbian affair then they started rumors that Reggie was having a homosexual affair with a student! I think they thought that they could break up our marriage. They didn't realize that Reggie and I had no secrets between us. We actually found some humor in the stories of our supposed sexual exploits. We would lie in bed together at night and compare notes on what stories we had heard. The kind of behavior we were being subject to was ridiculous.

Reggie rationalized that the teachers were like little kids not getting what they wanted, so they were acting out. I could find some humor in it, but I just didn't understand their vindictiveness. If they were so unhappy why didn't they just leave? After all, the school didn't owe them a living.

I saw the physical toll this was taking on Reggie. We were so close to perfection in the instruction of straight Chiropractic, but again, political wrangling and under the table deals were used to try and stop us. When we found out about the political nonsense we were heartbroken. We were even more heartbroken about the behavior from some of our supposed friends. It was like having your family suddenly turn on you. I told Reggie we'd find a way, we won't ever give up on keeping Chiropractic pure. Reggie had a dream of changing the world. He knew how great Chiropractic was, he just needed to find a way to deliver it to the people.

Everyone seemed to be against us. Reggie was killing himself, fighting battles on so many fronts, and many of them with supposed friends and straight Chiropractors. I finally persuaded Reggie that it was not worth it. It was one of the hardest decisions we ever made. Being so close, it was hard to let go.

When we decided to leave ADIO we got the last great insult. Reggie asked those who took over the school to pay him the salary he'd earned, but did not receive. He couldn't see funding a college that didn't want him. They did not send him the money. When he asked for an explanation, he was told that there needed to be an investigation into all financial activities between him and the college before they would release his money. The school acted like Reggie had embezzled money, and there were rumors that Reggie was dishonest.

At first we thought it was an honest accounting error, but when the money was withheld, we felt it was another insult. At that time Reggie received an invitation to speak in Australia, and several days after he left I received a call from a Chiropractor in Washington state. He'd heard that Reggie had to leave the country or he would've been thrown in jail for embezzling money from the college. He wanted to know if he could help me financially in any way.

The money issue was resolved many months later. We learned it was "close friends" who wanted to destroy our reputation, and when they couldn't hurt us with rumors of martial problems, they figured they could ruin our reputation by calling us crooks.

There was absolutely no basis in these false charges, and Reggie received his money. It was a bitter sweet victory. How happy can you be when you prove that the people you really trusted are trying to ruin you with false accusations about your integrity?

ADIO chugged along for a bit but it ultimately closed in 1995.   In retrospect, I feel that getting the school accredited in Pennsylvania would have been difficult with Reggie at the helm, because he was not open to compromise on any level when it came to Chiropractic. Obtaining CCE accreditation would have been next to impossible.

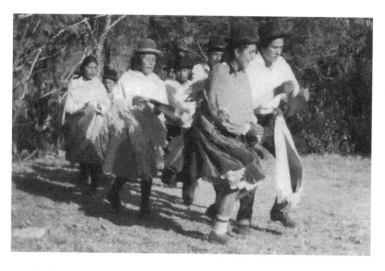

Before mission trips became fashionable, Reggie was adjusting the Quachua Indians of Peru. He not only adjusted them, but he stayed for 6 months and taught the native healers how to detect subluxation and adjust.

Chapter 15

Spinology - an answer to so many problems

After we left ADIO we realized that Chiropractic was in serious jeopardy. Reggie immediately sat down and thought of other ways that the principles of Chiropractic could live in a pure state, unhindered by politics and federal interference.

Reggie came up with Spinology. It was set up as a religion, so it was free from interference from political legislation. It was designed to get Chiropractic care to the masses. He really felt Chiropractic principles needed a place to be taught in their pure form, and taught in a way that didn't water down the importance of lifetime care.

Reggie wrote out all the terms and the Spinology program was started. Most of the first class were Europeans that had been sent by Chiropractors who were Sherman graduates practicing in Europe. These European students came to learn Spinology. They wanted the best we had to offer. Just like the early practitioners of Chiropractic, they had experienced the positive effects of spinal adjustments, and they fully embraced the concept. They didn't care about laws and accreditation. They were committed to bringing care to others.

We made every attempt to distinguish Spinology from Chiropractic. Instead of using terms like patients we called them "practice members." (This term has been adopted by many Chiropractors today). We used the term "vertabraile" for palpation. Reggie coined all the terms and wrote out all the tenets, as well as the educational requirements and course work. Because Spinology was registered as a church it was tax exempt, and because we were clear that it was not treating diseases or making diagnoses, we were free to concentrate on teaching technique and philosophy.

Students got basic anatomy and physiology. Our core palpation was muscle palpation or 'vertabraile". Our students became absolutely excellent adjusters and were rock solid with the philosophy.

The Sherman grads in Europe, Ireland, and Spain liked what they heard and saw from our students. They were excited to see students so solid and committed to helping others. After they saw the kind of practitioners Spinology produced, they talked us up and sent us students from all over. The European Chiropractors really promoted Spinology, and by word of mouth, Spinology really took off. Many of students from our first class are still in practice today.

Some began Spinology schools overseas. There's one school in Spain and another one in Ireland. Reggie was happy that Spinology was spreading. It was his dream that everyone have access to the Chiropractic tenets, no matter what it was called. Spinology was never about making money. In fact, it was purposefully setup to be virtually impossible to make much money running a Spinology school. The schools were easily affordable.

Reggie wanted people involved only for the betterment of other people. Spinology was formed to get people to promote the concept of what we believed in. However, Reggie eventually ended Spinology in the United States, because it had become a double-edged sword.

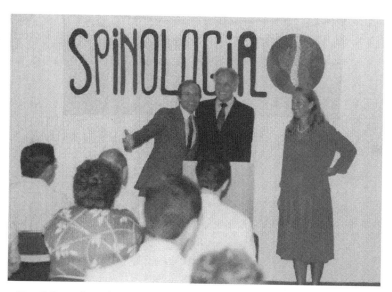

Dr. Miguel and Dr. Michelle Bolufer, Sherman graduates practicing in Spain as Spinologists. They and their family have become lifelong friends of the Golds. Spinology really took off – the public needed it, and the early practitioners were very enthusiastic.

It was easy to become a Spinologist, and we were getting applications from all over the world. The European schools were thriving and are still functioning today, but without offering an advanced degree. Because of this, it was difficult to attract the caliber of people he wanted in America. One thing Reggie could not compromise on was quality of practitioners. He felt the public deserved the best. Reggie would not teach adjusting or the tenets of Spinology to just anyone. He felt a moral obligation to make sure that person was going into practice for the right reasons.

After five years, it was with a heavy heart that Reggie stopped promoting Spinology. On many levels Spinology was a success. Reggie was absolutely passionate about the prospect of the correction of vertebral subluxation, and in doing so, changing the world. He felt it was his life's calling. He had to be involved with spreading the word.

Reggie felt that if he could get a large percentage of the people adjusted, not only would the world's population have better health, but the consciousness of the world would change. He saw correcting subluxation as a way to enhance the human race.

When he started Spinology, many people gave great support, but many long term friends and people in Chiropractic wrote us vicious letters. The hate mail was unbelievable. Reggie took most of it in stride, but no one could receive that kind of vitriol and be unaffected. Still, Reggie believed the detection and correction of subluxation was his life's work, whatever the personal price.

Thom Gelardi never abandoned Reggie. He understood Reggie's deep commitment to Chiropractic, and when Reggie stopped teaching Spinology, it was Thom who reached out with an olive branch and invited Reggie to speak. In Thom we had a kindred spirit in Chiropractic. Thom deeply believed in the same things we did, and when Sherman had money trouble, Reggie and I always backed him. I've witnessed precious few people that continue to put Chiropractic in front of their personal interests, and Thom Gelardi is one of those precious few.

I was at Sherman from 1974-78. Reggie was there from 1973-75, and went to ADIO in 1978. We realized our commitment to Chiropractic was larger than ourselves. We were being put to the test, and although we missed each other quite a bit, what we accomplished in Chiropractic has made up for it.

Chapter 16

On my own again

Gil Rodriguez was a teacher and student at Sherman. He came up with the idea to do a review class to prepare students for the national boards. We started with six weekends. Our first review had 53 students and only three passed.

I was an observer at a Part I national board exam that was administered at Sherman. There was a student from Palmer taking the exam at Sherman who had a large sheaf of rolled up papers, and when there was a break, he would look through them. He'd flip through them really fast. When I saw him going wild with these papers I thought, "What the heck is he doing?" On a break I asked him, and he showed me that he had all the old tests! I realized that almost all the questions he had were the same questions they just asked on the exam he took. Now I knew that some schools had old tests from which they were studying, and these questions were repeated on subsequent tests.

We had one more test to go, Microbiology. I called all the students in and then went through the microbiology questions and answers. No one failed Microbiology.

When I went over that exam I knew we were at a disadvantage, because we were teaching Chiropractic at Sherman. My pride was on the line. Sherman was the first new Chiropractic college in 25 years, and it was important to us that our students do well on the national board exams.

I decided I would do whatever it took to get these kids to pass the exam without giving up straight Chiropractic. I explained to the students that the test was just a hoop to jump through. They had to understand that it had nothing to do with Chiropractic.

Reggie got us in contact with students from many Chiropractic schools, and we got questions from previous tests. We gave our second review. We had 186 people and this time only three failed. We kept on giving reviews for Sherman students the entire time I was at Sherman. Slowly word got out about our review, and people began flying in from all over. Many of Life's C and D students came. They knew they didn't have a chance in the world at passing without help.

The first bunch of them arrived in a group of 20. They lived in my house for the week, in my basement. They were a great bunch of kids. They cleaned my house and even took care of my pool! We worked hard, and they all passed with great scores. They went back to Life and spread the word, and our review program really took off.

Our review started as a question and answer memorization, and as the test changed, we changed. I was always very weary of only giving questions and answers. I realized that the success of these people was in our hands, and I couldn't take that kind of responsibility lightly. I knew that in order to be successful we had to teach key concepts. If the students understood concepts, it didn't matter what they asked or how they asked it, our students could answer correctly!

Chapter 17

Culture shock

Living in South Carolina was difficult for Reggie and me. We were New Yorkers, and moving to South Carolina was a severe culture shock. I'll never forget my first trip to the grocery store. I stopped in for a few things and as I waited in a long line to pay for my groceries, there was a young girl working the cash register and talking to everyone in the line, like we have all the time in the world! I like movement. I don't like to stand around. They were talking about recipes for potatoes! Good grief, I have a thousand things to do and buying food took an hour.

On the more serious side, we had the ADIO emblem on our mail box, and somehow many people in town thought the sign indicated that we were devil worshippers. (It wasn't until years later that we learned that they were told this by a prominent Chiropractor in town who wanted us out).

People would drive through our property making noise. We'd call the police, but nothing happened. This went on for a quite a while. We thought if we ignored them, they'd lose interest and forget about us, but the opposite happened. They really ramped up their harassment. They started to drive by and shoot at our house or anything else that was an easy target on our property! It was so bad that we had to have students, mostly ex-military, protecting us.

One night I was sound asleep when suddenly I hear, "Get up with your hands up." Believe me, I fully woke up in a split second. I saw that Reggie was gone from the bed, so I looked out the window to see him holding a gun on a group of young men. He had them out of their car and was asking them what they wanted, and why they were harassing us.

"I want to know why you're doing this to us," he demanded. "I want you to come into the house and tell me why you are doing this!"

Well, this group came in and they told us their church leaders told them we were devil worshippers, and it was their duty to drive us out. We also found out that the police were in on it! We defused the situation by inviting the entire church to our house for a barbeque. Finally, after 18 months of terror, the harassment stopped.

I never felt welcome in South Carolina. The whole incident left us with a bad taste for the place. I was there for four years, two of which were hell, then two that were tolerable.

South Carolina was chosen because Lyle Sherman was Thom's mentor, and he wanted to be near Lyle. Thom was devoted to upper cervical.

The following article appeared in the Bucks County Courier Times on September 16, 1979.

Why were they shooting at Reggie Gold?
War among the Chiropractors

By Erik Larson
Courier Times Staff Writer

Shotguns once blazed around his house. Anonymous callers threatened his life. A South Carolina preacher branded him a devil worshipper.

It's all happened in the life of Reginald Gold, a Yardley chiropractor. A guru. A cult leader - his opponents have described him in these and stronger terms.

Gold, born in England, speaks with a soothing English accent. He is a tall man, with fluffy grey hair and dark complexion. He speaks in well-turned phrases without the little pauses that so often mar speech.

He and his wife, Irene, and their four dogs live in a spacious home on River Road in Yardley. Gold's love for Africa, where he has taught and traveled extensively, is reflected in the African statuary, the stools made from elephant feet, and the warm browns of his living room.

Reggie Gold is also at the center of battle between two groups of practitioners both claiming the name chiropractor and both more than willing to fight to keep it.

That's why people have said some terrible things about Reggie Gold. That's why rumors cluster around his name. Said a one-time associate, "There are a number of people who dislike Reggie Gold. It's not uncommon for them to attack him personally."

There are also his enemies who grudgingly admit the man has charisma. "He is dynamic," said one. "He is almost a guru."

In one camp are the "straights," chiropractors who believe you can only call yourself a chiropractor if you adhere to the original tenets of chiropractic - that it is a way of correcting subluxations of the human spine to maintain health and prevent disease. Subluxations, according to Daniel David Palmer, who founded chiropractic in 1895, are misalignments of spinal bones that impinge on the spinal cord.

No surgery

In the other camp are the "mixers," so-called because they supposedly mix chiropractic techniques with treatments and diagnostic procedures borrowed from medicine.

Neither is permitted by state law to prescribe drugs or do major surgery. In Oregon, one of the more permissive states, chiropractors can do very minor surgery, such as removing warts.

Gold believes the only chiropractor is a straight chiropractor. To venture into medical diagnosis, to pretend to be able to recognize diseases ranging from kidney disorders to is beyond the training of mixers, according to Gold.

But mixers want to become, part of the medical establishment,, he said, and they want to because they hunger for a piece of the huge dollar pie America has baked around its health care system.

In 1973, the mixers got a slice. A big slice. Chiropractors won federal recognition as legitimate practitioners when legislation gave them the right to bill Medicare and Medicaid for some of their services.

The Department of Health, Education and Welfare did not approve.

HEW, several years before, had criticized inadequacies in chiropractic education, and chiropractors' poor diagnostic skills. While conceding that some chiropractic skills could be beneficial to persons suffering joint pain, the agency concluded chiropractic services should not be covered by Medicare.

Clear danger

In 1974, mixers got another slice. The U.S. Office of Education approved the Council on Chiropractic Education as an accrediting institution. The CCE was fathered by the American Chiropractic Association, the parent organization for mixers. Now chiropractic schools could accredit themselves and be eligible for financial aid from federal sources.

96

By encouraging chiropractors to adopt and teach medical techniques, Gold charges, these acts moved mixers closer to becoming a public hazard.

Even for specialists, diagnosis is a guessing game, Gold said. For others, even more so. "Chiropractors cannot diagnose effectively. To pretend that they can is a clear and present danger to the public .health."

The Office of Education's approval of the CCE escalated the battle. Straight chiropractors accuse the CCE of trying to suppress the straights by setting academic standards they could not philosophically accept.

Mixers deny the charge. They say they are enlightened practitioners trying to bring chiropractic out of the dark ages.

Last spring the Council on Chiropractic Education went back to the Office of Education to renew its accrediting status. Gold testified at the hearing as president of the Federation of Straight Chiropractic Organizations, representing a variety of straight associations.

Gold charged that the initial approval by the Office of Education "has been used to the detriment of the entire educational process in chiropractic, and above all to the detriment of its consumers, the public at large."

"To pretend a chiropractor in four years can accomplish what a physician learns in 12 years is an insult to the medical profession," Gold testified.

"It was that testimony that really brought the wrath of God down on me," said Gold in an interview last week.

CCE approval

Transcripts of the hearing show testimony from both camps split and
confused the review committee. Instead of granting the usual three-year renewal, this committee voted 9 to 2 to approve the CCE for only one year, during which the philosophies and allegations of the groups could be studied.

In an unprecedented move, Ernest Boyer, Commissioner of Education, overruled the committee and granted a-three year renewal.

The wrath of mixers has been directed at Gold for nearly two decades.

He came to the United States from London in 1950, and worked as an antique dealer.

In 1954, Gold went to a chiropractor. If a man can be born again in a chiropractor's office, he was. "What he said to me made so much sense - nothing in health had made that much sense to me before."

Gold enrolled in the Palmer College of Chiropractic in Davenport, Iowa, the "fountainhead" of chiropractic.

In 1961 Gold became an instructor - and later a dean - at the Columbia Institute of Chiropractic, since renamed the New York College of Chiropractic. In 1963, he was fired by Ernest Napolitano, the school's president, for what Napolitano says were philosophical reasons.

Cheating charged

Gold set up practice in Spring Valley, New York. He built a profitable practice on patients' donations. He never charged a fee, believing that a price should not be put his kind of health-preserving skills.

In 1972 he applied for a chiropractor's license in South Carolina where he planned to establish the Sherman College of Chiropractic in Spartanburg. He expected the board of chiropractic examiners to approve his license based on a reciprocal relationship with New York.

Gold was extensively interviewed. "Grilled," he said. Later he received a letter stating his request was refused, that New York and South Carolina did not reciprocate.

He sat for the exams; three months later he was told he had failed. "I know damn well I didn't fail," he said. He asked to review the tests and grading. The examiners wrote back stating he hadn't really failed, but had cheated and would not receive a license.

A South Carolina Attorney General's investigation of the cheating apparently reached no conclusions, and case was closed in 1978, according to Marsha Wright of the attorney general's staff.

Gold had not taken the board's charge lightly. He sued on the grounds the board was unconstitutional, that it could not judge him because it did not represent the public and the straights; that it consisted only of mixers.

A South Carolina Supreme Court judge agreed, and ordered the board dis-banded. During this period Gold came in for a real dose of holy wrath. A local preacher, allegedly at the urging of other chiropractors, spat hell and damnation at Gold, proclaiming him and his followers devil worshippers.

Shots fired

That brought the locals driving across Gold's lawn in the night, firing shotguns and narrowly missing at least one of his students.

Gold stayed on to help the school get started then came north, smack into more trouble in New York. There the New York Board of Chiropractic examiners took him to task for flamboyant and misleading advertising.

The board suspended his license for four months, staying three of them. It didn't matter. Gold had already left the state.

Gold came to Bristol Township to set up the ADIO Institute of Straight Chiropractic. It's motto - chiropractic without compromise.

In August 1978, the ADIO Institute, now in the George Clymer Elementary School building on Sunset Avenue, sued the Bucks County and Pennsylvania Chiropractic societies charging them with carrying out a smear campaign against ADIO. That ease is pending.

Just last week Gold testified in yet another suit. And for an unlikely organization - the American Medical Association which has called chiropractic "an unscientific cult whose practitioners lack the training and background to diagnose and treat human disease."

The mixers, according to Gold, are suing the AMA for violating anti-trust laws by restraining their practice. Gold said he would testify that the AMA is not "restraining the practice of medicine but the improper practice of medicine by mixers."

Gold resigned from ADIO August 4, again refusing to compromise. Some faculty members apparently wanted a salary, something he believes teachers of chiropractic should never receive.

With family members controlling the board of trustees, he could have kept control of the school. But he said he could not

99

work in "that atmosphere of disharmony and distrust" and turned the presidency over to Dr. Joseph Strauss.

Gold will go on fighting, and will probably continue to draw controversy.

"If you don't try to change the world, everything else is Mickey Mouse," Gold is fond of saying. "It's fun to change the world."

Chapter 18

Irene takes charge

My board review company went from a local affair to a large scale business fairly quickly. I continued to do national board reviews, but when I left Sherman, I was told I couldn't continue teaching the program there. I guess people at Sherman thought I would poach students from them and send them to ADIO. This is something I would never have done! They just didn't know me and the kind of person I was, or how devoted I was to Chiropractic. Regardless, the students demanded I come back to Sherman, so I did.

As I got busier and put more time into the review class, I decided I couldn't sit around waiting for students to come to me. I needed to bring this great information to the students. The class had developed into something really special, and people really needed the service. We had the key concepts down, so it didn't matter what questions were asked, our students could answer, and they could understand why the answer was correct.

When I left Sherman, I decided to form a corporation in Pennsylvania where I lived and taught at ADIO. I decided we would cover three colleges, New York Chiropractic College, Sherman, and Life. Since Gil Rodrigues graduated and went in to practice, I needed a new partner, so I approached an extremely bright student at Sherman, and he agreed to work with me.

To grow, I needed a loan for $5,000. I incorporated my business in 1978, and that $5,000 loan was money we really needed. The bank turned me down, and told me that my husband had to cosign. I explained that it wasn't his business, it was my business. The bank manager, a "man", patiently explained to me the bank would not lend money to women! And this was 1978! I would not give in. I wanted that loan in my name because it was my company, and it was my responsibility to pay back the money. Finally I used Reggie's car as collateral to get the $5,000.

Six weeks later I paid them back. Then six months later my brilliant partner wanted out. He said I was going nowhere! He wanted $5,000 to be bought out. I had to go through the same routine again with the bank and again I gave Reggie's car over as collateral and I got the $5,000. It took six weeks and again I paid them back.

After that, we really took off. I had 500 people sign up for the class. Now the bank was calling me asking how much money I wanted. I was never so happy to tell them "I don't want a dime from you!"

From then on all our classes were big. We branched out and began going to five schools, and then it became really huge. We never forgot who we were serving, and that our end goal was to get Chiropractors out in the field so that they could practice Chiropractic.

Dr. Bernie Diskin called me in 1980. He was a Chiropractor that had been out of school for a long time. He'd been a big promoter of Parker Seminars in Australia, and he wanted to come back to the United States and practice, but he kept failing the test. He asked if I would come out and teach the basic science for the California exam. I told him I didn't know much about the California boards, but I'd do my best to get them through. We made a deal for a group of ten people. I figured I needed ten people to meet my expenses.

Five days before I was to leave Bernie called me and told me that they only had 3 people signed up and those three were willing to pay the entire amount to cover the seven empty seats. I told him that was not acceptable to me. I didn't want anyone to have to pay extra. I told them I'd come out and give the class for the three that signed up.

When I flew out to California, seventeen people showed up at the class! Everyone in the group had failed the test at least once before, and one person had failed sixteen times over an eight year period. I'll never forget this one joker. He stood up on the first day of class before I had even said a word and announced, "I don't even know why I'm here, this is a rip off."

I knew his attitude could ruin the entire class, and there was no way I was going to let one person stand in the way of sixteen people passing, so I told him in front of everyone, "You can have your money back, get out! I don't need your money! And I don't need your attitude!"

He calmed right down and then he apologized. I'm glad he stayed, because he and everyone else passed that test, including the chronic failure. The person who'd failed sixteen times came to me after the test in tears. He told me there were only three questions he didn't know the answer to. The reward in teaching is "helping the people." The money is secondary.

It was during this review that I got the idea to start adding more time to cover the information from every conceivable angle. One woman missed a class due to a death in her family. She asked if I could stay after class and catch her up on the work she'd missed. I figured the whole class could use a review, so instead of going our normal 8am to 5pm, I decided to go until 8pm. It worked, so well that the next day I went from 8am to 11pm. It was a full immersion system. They couldn't help but pass after being exposed to 12 to 14 hours of information per day!

The key was to start very simple. You wouldn't believe some of the easy concepts that people get confused over early on, and when they never get corrected, it throws off the rest of their education. One person would often muster the courage to ask a "simple" question, and then I'd ask anyone in the class to give the answer, and absolutely no one knew it.

We have some major problems in our educational system. Teachers have to become more aware of students' needs. We have to make sure that all students get a good understanding of basic concepts so they are solid in their education from the first day onward. I am forever grateful to those confused students who taught me the way to teach people. I got the best education from those people.

There are so many elementary questions that need to be cleared up early so that people can understand. I searched for those basic questions that never got cleared up, and once we got those concepts explained, these students soared.

My class was designed to get people that had absolutely no chance to pass to succeed. At that time we were only teaching information for Parts I and II of the national boards, and then I found out many students were still failing the clinical part of the California exam. Dr. Chris Kent was working for me then, so we decided to start teaching x-ray and clinical material as well. There was no way we were going to work so hard on the basic sciences and not have these students get a license. That was unacceptable to me.

There was an organization in California at this time that was just doing a California review, and they only did the clinical part. We went into competition with them, and after a year they closed down. We had between 300 and 350 students for the California boards, which was a lot better than our original three!

Chapter 19

Why?

In the beginning, board review classes emphasized memorization. Then the boards made a major change in 1978. They stopped using just Chiropractic concepts and really went medical. In a way, they didn't ask harder questions, they just made the exam confusing. It seemed like they were upset that Sherman grads had the top scores throughout all the schools in the United States, and we were said to be light on education at Sherman!

We knew for sure that we were teaching the most about Chiropractic, and so did those administering the board exams. It upset them that we were academically one of the top schools.

After 1978, I really felt the pressure of the politics of the profession and the board. I was no longer welcome on campuses, and I was even banned from some of them. At Cleveland Chiropractic in Los Angeles I was escorted off campus, and not allowed to set foot on the property without a scheduled appointment. I was also banned at National College in Lombard. I went into the book store and was detained by security for over an hour. They said I needed an appointment to be on campus. They didn't want any part of me.

The politicians of the national board put a lot of pressure on the colleges to ban of me because they felt our teaching was too good, and it was giving the students who attended our review a big advantage in passing the boards.

Even Sid Williams didn't allow me on Life's campus. I am sure some of this had to do with Reggie, and some of it had to do with all the strong personalities. I just wish we could have all realized that we were all working toward the same goal in the straight Chiropractic community.

We allowed the medical mixer crew in Chiropractic to fragment us straights into ever smaller subgroups. The tests are basically medical examinations which do not reflect our Chiropractic knowledge at all. The only test that even comes remotely close to having anything to do with Chiropractic is the Part IV-Technique exam. The profession has to wake up and realize that they are testing us as if we are going to practice medicine, not Chiropractic. The schools have been forced to shift focus to medicine in order for students to pass these exams, instead of focusing on the important Chiropractic information.

I did my best to try to tell people that the exam has nothing to do with Chiropractic. After the reviews, many students were excited and wanted more time with me, to see if they could understand Chiropractic, and I mean *real* Chiropractic. It is such a monumental shame that many students aren't being educated in Chiropractic, nor are they given a proper medical education. Effectively, they can't practice in either profession.

I've never understood why on earth any Chiropractic college would want to give a medical education. There are so many paths towards a life in medicine. There are medical schools, nursing schools, medical technician programs and even physician's assistant programs. So why on earth would you go to a Chiropractic college to learn that stuff when there are so many other places to become involved with medicine, and only a few places to learn Chiropractic? Chiropractic is absolutely separate and distinct from medicine. We are not an alternative to medicine, nor are we a branch or off shoot. Chiropractic stands completely separate in its ideals and values about health and its potential.

I am proud to say that even in teaching a class to pass a required medical exam, we have been able to spread the message about straight Chiropractic. We let the students know that the tests are just hoops to jump through, something to pass and then forget about, because they have **absolutely nothing to do with the practice of Chiropractic.**

Chapter 20

Commitment

Reggie and Irene spent 25 years in promoting Chiropractic. Reggie had 13 years in active practice, and he taught in three Chiropractic colleges: Columbia, Sherman and ADIO. He was involved in starting two Chiropractic colleges, Sherman and ADIO. He lectured in every state in America, and gave Chiropractic talks on every continent on earth. He was on radio, television and he spoke to millions about the benefits of Chiropractic care.

He revitalized PACE, the patients' organization that promoted Chiropractic. He inspired thousands of people to begin Chiropractic careers, and inspired hundreds of thousands to try Chiropractic care. He gave thousands of public talks in every imaginable situation, in gyms auditoriums, restaurants, colleges, churches, synagogues, and on street corners, and in Chiropractors offices throughout the world.

He explained Chiropractic philosophy to students, Chiropractors, medical personnel, governors and anyone else you can imagine. He helped start a new accrediting agency, SCASA, to accredit straight schools rather than use the CCE, which in Reggie's view, had a clear goal of dismantling Chiropractic.

He was a representative of the ICA, beginning in college working with B.J. Palmer, and then as a state representative. When he felt the ICA no longer supported

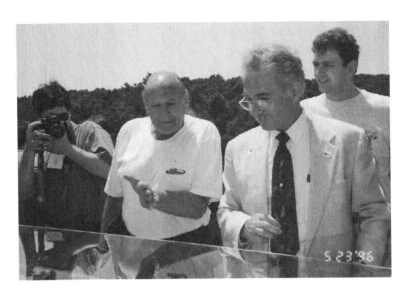

Reggie and Thom "looking it over"

the practice of straight Chiropractic, he wrote the bylaws and started a new Chiropractic organization, FSCO (now called IFCO), to represent Chiropractic into the future.

This is only a partial list of Reggie's achievements. After 25 years of this kind of activity, most people would take a well-deserved break. Reggie and Irene had the financial wherewithal to fade quietly into retirement and spend the rest of their lives in each other's company, living wherever and doing whatever they chose. But Reggie and Irene chose another 25 years in Chiropractic. They never missed a beat, and plunged headlong into doing what they do best: promoting Chiropractic.

Reggie started lecturing again. First the offers came in slowly, but then as people heard his message, requests for speaking engagements came from all over the world. Irene's board review program continued to grow. As

Irene's reputation grew, she became sought after by the same colleges that used to ban her.

When Reggie spoke, he promoted Sherman. His affinity for Sherman and Thom Gelardi never wavered. He felt that Sherman students and Sherman Chiropractic College had that something special, that extra bit that made them special. As more people heard Reggie speak, the demand grew for his Chiropractic talks, his patient education lectures, his debates with medical people, and in general anything Reggie said.

In response to the demand for his work, the website www.reggiegold.com was born. It is a website that has the complete collection of Reggie's greatest talks. The one speech that most agree is Reggie at his finest is "Valley of the Blind", which was first given in 1972, at Palmer College, before 1,500 people. It is really something special to hear Reggie's eloquent speech, and sit on the edge of your seat during his dramatic pauses. It is a powerful message that has helped enlighten Chiropractors and lay people alike. We are fortunate that it is available on CD.

Chapter 21

50 years of service

It is impossible to document all the achievements of Irene and Reggie Gold. In a span of 50 years they have touched the hearts of countless people.

Irene worked alongside Reggie and at times took the lead. She founded and ran the largest board review program in the world. She is still teaching today. She has taught at both Sherman and ADIO, served as an administrator at Sherman (as Dean of Academics), and has spoken to people all over the world about Chiropractic care. Irene has given countless patient education talks, and motivated people from all over the world to become Chiropractors.

She holds multiple degrees, RN, BS, MA, and DC. This educational achievement alone staggers the mind. It is almost inconceivable that all this education was earned while working full time and promoting Chiropractic.

One thing the Golds both agreed on is that the most important thing they've done is to be in love with one another, followed by their love of Chiropractic, which they've tirelessly shared with others. Being involved with Chiropractic has forced their private life to be public. They spent many long weeks and months away from one another while giving talks, founding colleges and promoting Chiropractic. In their over 50 year marriage, their devotion to each other and to Chiropractic has never wavered.

Reggie passed away on March 24, 2012. Irene was by his side, in death as she was in life. There is profound sadness, and the loss of his companionship is difficult, but there is an understanding that death is as natural as life.

We cling to life's beauty and long to see our dreams fulfilled. Reggie passed without regrets and without bitterness, as he had an unending love and passion for his wife, and for Chiropractic. He left with the hope that the world and Chiropractic were better off than when he arrived. He was gladdened and hopeful that straight Chiropractic was picking up adherents. He was so pleased IFCO experiencing a resurgence in recent years, and that young Chiropractors were picking up where he left off.

Reggie passed, having lived life well, because his life was dedicated to serving people, and a cause larger than himself.

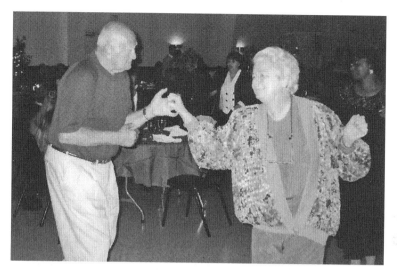

Reggie and Irene "cutting the rug"

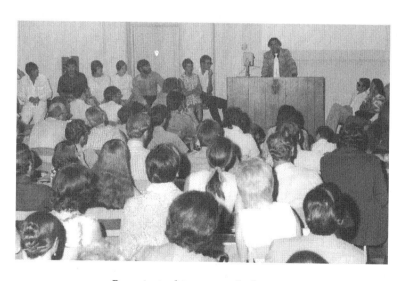

Reggie in his natural element

Irene Gold, to me, is the true expression of altruism that is often talked about by many, but practiced by few. I can remember countless times watching her teach from the crack of dawn until the wee hours of the night, until her voice was virtually gone, but never her enthusiasm. Never once did it seem that there was anything more important than helping that person in front of her at that moment in time.

25 years later she is still going with the same intensity, enabling more Chiropractors to get out and help more sick people. Thank you for all you did for me. Thank you from all of my patients, and most all of thank you for seeing something greater in me than I knew about.

-Marc Schwartz

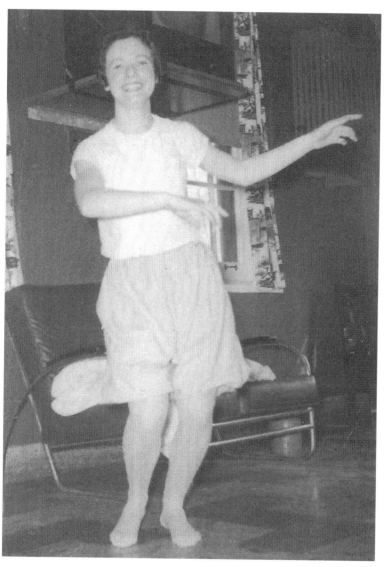

Irene happy with life

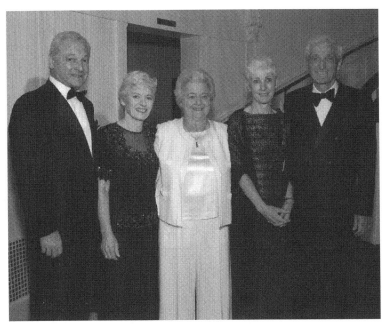

Richard Siemens, Marion Glim, Irene Gold,
Carrie Trust, and Walter Siemens

Chapter 22

The end is the beginning

Judd Nogrady

I was fortunate to spend much of my childhood with my grandfather. Grandpa was still youthful and highly energetic in his late 80's. Much of his zest for life came from his one maxim, "Succeed not for yourself, but so that the next guy who comes along can have it a little easier." Before I met Irene, I thought that there wasn't a finer individual in the world than my grandfather. His mentality of "leave the world a better place than you found it" and his unstoppable drive made him a powerful force.

In Irene we find another person cut from that fine, tough, resilient cloth. It is my honor to know her and a larger honor to work with her. I was always taught that to be truly successful in life you had to have great friends, family, and a mission that was larger than yourself. Irene Gold measures up to this, and beyond, in all categories.

As I interviewed people for this book, countless ones told me stories of the lengths Irene had gone to help them. "Above and beyond" and "loving and caring" became words spoken over and over. For Irene, above and beyond and love and caring is a way of life. Chiropractic is her passion, and a life of service to Chiropractic is her trademark.

As Irene spoke of her retirement, she quickly outlined her "retirement" plans. These include working as an instructor for her company Irene Gold Reviews, with her business partner John Donofrio. She moved to Florida as the first step in this retirement plan. The move to Florida, to be close to her family, has been planned for some time.

Richard (brother) and his wife Carole, and their children Allen, Scott, Robert, and Rebecca, all live in Florida.

Joy (sister-in-law, widow of brother Walter) and their son Ronald, live in Florida, son Paul in California, and daughter Amy in New York.

Marion (sister) and her husband Ben, are in Florida, and their son Stephen in California and daughter Rachel in Pennsylvania.

Carrie (sister), and her husband Allan live in Florida, and their children Howard and Randi live in New Jersey.

It is a point of pride that all of these nieces and nephews are college graduates.

Once retirement has been established, Irene will be giving private tutoring to those individuals and small groups of Chiropractors that need a little extra help. She also plans on traveling extensively while attending numerous Chiropractic functions. When Irene speaks of retirement, she has the same animation in her body and that same spark in her eyes as when I first saw her demonstrating the different "walks people have" with different medical conditions during my Part II board review program.

When she leans in close to tell me an off the record story, it is with the same smile she had when someone asked the same question for the tenth time after a 12 hour marathon tutoring session.

Irene has managed to capture that something special that separates Chiropractic and Chiropractors from other people and other professions: a pure love for the world and the people in it. It is my greatest honor and pleasure to call Irene my friend, and Chiropractic my profession.

All my best to you fellow Chiropractors. May your life bring joy to others, for then you will be rich beyond the greatest measure.

-Judd Nogrady

Irene Gold

In writing this book, I feel I have to acknowledge those people who took the time and trouble to help out when Reggie was reaching the end of his life.

Reggie was admitted to the hospital on January 1, 2012, because he could not breathe well enough with the oxygen supply we had at home. He was treated for congestive heart failure with drugs to alleviate the fluid in his lungs. This treatment caused him to go into kidney failure. After a few days, when it was obvious that medical treatment was not for him, he opted to discontinue all medical treatment and be taken home. I asked the doctors how long they thought he would survive without their care, and they told me that at home he would not last longer than a few days.

At this point I called Dr. Jim Dubel of New Beginnings seminars in New Jersey, to let him know what was happening so he could make the Chiropractic community aware of the situation. And then came the miracle. Thousands of people responded on Facebook, and hundreds of emails were received from those who were close friends, and from others whom we didn't even know. Every day I brought Reggie a new set of emails, and each day he got stronger, so that he didn't need the oxygen supply as often. Those emails kept him alive for almost three months. I want to thank everyone who sent them.

There was a time that I needed to leave to teach a class, and asked Reggie if he would be okay without me. I would find people to stay with him while I was away. Many offered to come and stay, but he only chose those with whom he would feel most comfortable.

Kimberly Goreham, though not a Chiropractor, is very strong Chiropractic advocate and educator. Reggie chose her, and she came from California to be with him. Dr. Judy Campanale, a local Chiropractor in Pennsylvania, who has been a strong supporter of the straight Chiropractic movement, was also chosen by Reggie. Dr. Michael Holt, a graduate of Life University, kindly offered to stay for a few days, so I picked him. Ines Bolufer Laurentie, daughter of Miguel and Michelle Bolufer, are all Chiropractors from Spain. Ines spent her years in college living with us in Pennsylvania, and has become part of our family. She and her husband Thomas, and their children Sarah and Lukas, spent time with Reggie in the hospital and then came to be with me in the last few hours of Reggie's life. Reggie picked her to stay with him.

I also wish to thank Bryan Amaral, a close friend to Reggie, who came to the hospital and stayed for the night shift, so he could be watched 24 hours a day. I also wish to thank Dr. Sharon Gorman, Dr. Joe Strauss, Dr. Tom Gregory, Dr. and Mrs. Jim Dubel, Dr. David Scheiner, and Dr. Brian Kelly, who came to our home during those last few months to adjust Reggie or just to sit and talk to him.

This profession actually became my family in time of need. Thank you all.

Letters

In writing and researching our book we received boxes of letters, news clipping, magazine articles, and photo, video and audio recordings. We have read, reread, listened, and watched them all, learning all the while.

Some of the many submissions are included here in the book as we received them, most with no edits or very slight alterations in spelling. Our hope is that you enjoy and savor the hearts, minds and souls that so many in our profession possess. We hope you feel the love, hope and courage they have, and may it help you to tell the message "just one more time."

All the best to you,

Irene Gold

Judd Nogrady

CHIROPRACTORS

Dear Irene,

It was a great pleasure hearing from you this morning. You were on my mind all weekend and I was delighted to hear your voice and to know that you were concerned about my Part IV results. Needless to say, you and the gang more than adequately prepared me for the exam (605 big ones!).

I had never taken a review before this one because of my misconception of what the reviews were. While they are indeed, training sessions to help one pass the specific exam for which they are intended, they are also incredible teaching tools to help make better doctors.

Palmer West did a great job in providing me with an education to enable me to practice Chiropractic. Irene Gold and Associates solidified much of that education by creatively reinforcing concepts and procedures. I had a blast in your course, and would not have traded all those hours with you and Donofrio for anything.

You made the class fun, motivating, and educational and did a phenomenal job in preparing us for what could have been a brutal experience. Donofrio was spectacular! He kept our interest, utilizing his unique ability to read students and to know who needs what. He is a true and brilliant master that I will remember for the rest of my life.

You kept me entertained and interested throughout the entire review and it was truly a pleasure to learn by your methods. If there is anything I can do to help you and your associates, please feel free to contact me at any time, and I will gladly drop whatever I am doing to help you. I hope that I have conveyed to you my deepest appreciation for your unselfish effort. I could never have done this without you.

Sincerely,

Jack M. Bourla, DC

Redwood City, CA

Founding member of Schübel Vision Seminars

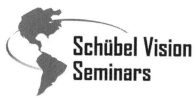

www.schubelvision.com

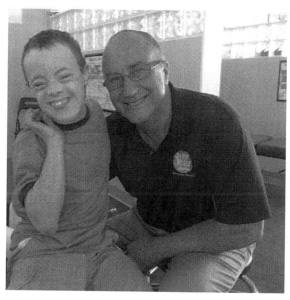

Jack Bourla with a practice member

The famous BJ quote, "You never know how far reaching…" could never be more appropriate in my life with respect to Irene Gold. I was an excellent Chiropractic student, graduating top in my class. I did extremely well on national boards Parts I-III. When it came time to take Part IV, I did not want to risk failing the boards. Doing so would mean delaying my license by six months, and six months meant a great deal to me. So I enrolled in Irene Gold's Part IV review class.

She was remarkable. She actually made preparing for the mundane fun. We learned, we laughed, we prepared. I knew the stuff cold. I was ready for anything they threw at us. Irene knew it. We had a rapport. She knew I was very prepared.

Friday afternoon of the dreaded weekend came and it was my turn to take the x-ray portion of the exam. The students are placed in a dark room with 10 stations of films and questions related to the films. Each station is timed. When the examiners say "go", the students each go to their assigned station and begin. When I arrived at my first station, I asked myself "Is this a joke?" "Is this a human X ray?" I panicked. I couldn't make out what I was looking at and the timer went off…time for Station 2. But I had not yet answered the questions for Station 1.

I went to Station 2 thinking about the questions for Station 1. I did my best to answer Station 2 and tried to answer Station 1 with the time I had remaining. The timer went off to go to Station 3. I was still thinking about Station 1 and now even Station 2. It continued for 10 Stations and I thought I was a dead man.

After the exam, we were herded to a holding room. During the cattle march, I spoke with another student who did not take the review course. He said it was a breeze. I told him I failed miserably and was not going to take the remainder of the exam. Somehow, that information got back to Irene and she called me at home that night and asked me what I thought of the exam. I told her I failed. She told me I was "crazy" and to not "be silly." If I failed, she reasoned, everyone else failed. She insisted I take the remainder of the test.

I listened to her and did. My scores came back. I killed all sections of Part IV. She was right. Had I not listened to her, I would have bailed from the exam and delayed receiving my license by 6 months.

Here is the amazing thing: I ran into Irene and Reggie Gold at a conference 15 years later and she stopped me in the hallway and recanted the entire story, verbatim, as though it had just happened. She remembers everything and everyone. Her memory is unparalleled. She remembers stories from 40 years ago, in great detail. She is an unbelievable treasure to the profession. Her commitment to the students is so remarkable that everyone she touches benefits.

And that guy who bragged about the x-ray section being a breeze: he failed Part IV. He should've taken the review course with me.

Jack M. Bourla, DC

Redwood City, CA

www.providencechiropracticcenter.com

Reggie Gold, D.C. was the very first person I met in 1973 when I arrived, at nearly midnight, at the Greenville-Spartanburg Airport in South Carolina. I had flown from Paris France to JFK in New York, to La Guardia and then Spartanburg. I did not speak any English, and this jovial man with long side burns, extravagant clothing and rhinestone jewels walked up to me with a grin on his face and said, "Bonjour, you must be Arno." I breathed a sigh of relief, as I was the only passenger left in the airport, and I had nothing with me but the phone number of Thom Gelardi, D.C., the President to be of Sherman College of Chiropractic. The next thing I knew we were flying in Reggie's Citroen-Maserati, out of the airport, skidding through most of the on ramp curve of I-85 North, and launched on to the Highway. I thought, "This is a man after my own heart!"

Reggie was an amazing teacher. He had a way of conveying Chiropractic philosophical building blocks in depth, then opening up the class for questions. As eager students, we would raise our hands, excited to have the answer. Countless times we were way off, and Reggie would crush us in such a way that we would not dare to come out of our hole for quite some time. This way of teaching forced us to investigate, inquire, and dig deeply into Chiropractic philosophy, in the hope of emerging with a correct answer. I believe that it is mainly because of Reggie Gold that I acquired a rock solid foundation in Chiropractic principles and philosophy.

Another instance sticks in my mind to this day, because it affected my speaking career. Reggie invited me to come to a student recruitment program in Virginia Beach. Reggie was giving a talk to inspire prospective students. When we arrived at the venue and were about to step into the conference room, he turned to me and said; "Arno, you give the talk tonight." I thought I would die right here and then. This experience showed me how much I could deliver, though totally unprepared, and in spite of extreme perspiration, dried mouth and the feeling I was going to lose my bowels!

Over the years I stayed connected to Reggie, with multiple encounters on various speaking platforms. I also felt the need and duty to write to him from time to time and express my deep gratitude for his amazing mentoring and teaching influence. To date, Reggie remains in my heart and mind as an icon and one of the most influential Chiropractor of our century.

Arno Burnier, D.C.

Durango, CO

www.cafeoflife.com, www.zeechi.com, www.mcqi.org

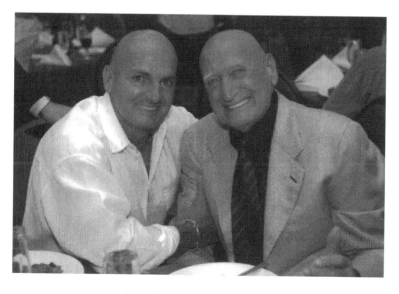

Arno Burnier and Reggie

Dear Irene,

It is about time that the profession recognize you, you have done so much for so long, all hidden in the background of Reggie. I am so grateful for you being my teacher at Sherman, for your humor, good laughs and bright mind. You infused me with passion and inspired me. You also "saved" me from real trouble when I was dealing with ways to keep myself afloat financially as a student. I am so glad that our lives intersected so often and that I could always hug you to express my gratitude.

LOVE, LOVE, LOVE,

Arno Burnier, D.C.

Durango, CO

www.cafeoflife.com, www.zeechi.com, www.mcqi.org

Dear Reggie,

I first saw and heard you speak about 35 years ago at a Garden State Chiropractic Society meeting. I was a student at Columbia Institute of Chiropractic. Your message was so different than what I heard in school. You helped form my foundation for practicing principled Chiropractic for the last 32 years. I was honored to speak on the same platform as you recently in Peru and at New Beginnings. So many have weakened their resolve over the years, but not you.

Thank you for holding the line, never wavering, and being an inspiration for truth.

With much love and gratitude,

Bradley S. Rausch, D.C.

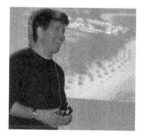

Bradley S. Rausch

Dr. Reggie Gold is a true Chiropractic legend who saved my Chiropractic career. Reggie came to Windsor, Ontario, Canada to speak at the Knights of Columbus when I was attending the university studying kinesiology.

At that time, I knew I wanted to be a Chiropractor. I was working as a Chiropractic assistant, running between 5 different rooms using ultrasound, muscle stimulation current, flexion distraction tables, hot wax, and hot and cold packs. After I was done, the Chiropractor would come in and talk to the patient, asking about their pain, how their family was doing, and discuss the latest sports game that was on the night before. Sometimes they would get an adjustment. When Reggie Gold came to town we closed the office and the whole staff had to go hear him speak.

Needless to say, I left a different person than when I walked in. He brought purpose to the practice of Chiropractic and saved me from a lifetime of rehabilitation.

By listening to Reggie's recordings I graduated as a principled Chiropractor from a school environment focused on rehabilitation. I listened to Reggie's "Starting a Chiropractic Practice" recordings to help open my practice the right way. I listened to "The Philosophy" to keep myself rooted in what I should have been taught in college.

Thank you Dr. Reggie Gold for making me realize that Chiropractic is more powerful than the waves coming out of an ultrasound head, and that I can connect with patients through the principled Chiropractic message, and not through talking about sports.

Now my motto is "Get Principled, Stay Principled". At the Solid Foundation Family Chiropractic Clinic Dr. Reggie Gold will always be a part of our Solid Foundation and has helped me stay principled.

Dr. Brock Van Dyke, DC

Waterdown, Ontario, Canada

www.solidfoundation.ca

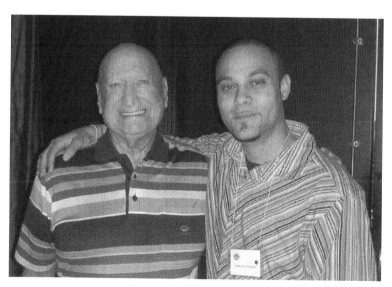

Reggie with Brock Van Dyke

Hello Reggie and Irene,

You do not know me, but you do - you have raised me in Chiropractic. My name is Larry Silverstein. I have been a Chiropractor for 31 years in Watertown, NY.

Irene, you helped my wife Becky Keshmiri pass her boards. In doing such, she in her exuberant passion for the principle has helped transform many lives. I am now 57 years old. I grew up in Paramus, NJ, and had many adjustments by Joe Donofrio.

My dad started us as a family getting adjusted in about 1960 on a regular basis. It was one of a handful of things we did consistently as a family. You were the influence and backdrop to all of this. I play your tapes to my team during our training sessions. I love you Reggie.

Feel my soft palpable embrace,

Larry Silverstein

www.watertownchiropractor.com

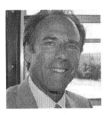

Larry Silverstein

Dr. Gold,

I just wanted to send an email to say thank you for helping me successfully prepare for my Florida boards. You did an excellent job in preparing us. I had been out of school since 1994, and felt I would never be ready for the boards. I was overwhelmed my first day of the review. I had only vague memories of most of the information presented those first few days. I have been teaching for the last four years, so my Chiropractic skills were diminished. It all came together for me the last few days of the review.

I kept saying to myself "this woman knows what she is doing" because you have helped thousands of people pass boards. So I went over everything you said would be there, and eliminated things you said wouldn't. When I walked in to the exam I was nervous but I kept my composure, took my time, and went through the process you had drilled us on over three weeks.

It was like reading a road map. I didn't add anything or delete anything. I followed the script as it was given and the answers began to flow. The things I learned in the review and during my schooling came back to me. I was even able to get through the soft tissue technique because I just made the muscle do the opposite to stretch it out. Thank you so much, you have helped me through all of my boards.

Eternally Grateful,

Dr. Judy

Reggie and Irene,

We continue to send positive thoughts to you both on this journey. Know that we love and appreciate you both, and also know how much you both mean to us as a Chiropractic couple. We "sharpened our teeth", so to speak, at your home on Ellish Parkway in Spring Valley, in preparation for what has become an incredible life of helping people by practicing straight, unadulterated Chiropractic.

Ingrained in our memory are the many weekends spent sitting on those uncomfortable steps at your home, but attaining an understanding of Chiropractic philosophy that to date is still unsurpassed. Because of you, our vision had been expanded to caring for literally hundreds of people a day (not as many as you Reggie...I'm still jealous of that...only kidding) and educating them to a different way of looking at life.

Thanks again from the bottom of our hearts, and know that you will always be in our thoughts.

Much Love,

Bobby and Evelyn Tarantino

Dear Irene,

To the woman behind the legend, know that we love and appreciate you for what you continue to give to the our profession. We have always held you and Reggie in the highest regard and we will forever be grateful to you for helping us become the Chiropractic family that we are. Both Evelyn and I would not be as successful in Chiropractic without your influence and for this we are continually grateful.

Love Evelyn and Bob Tarantino

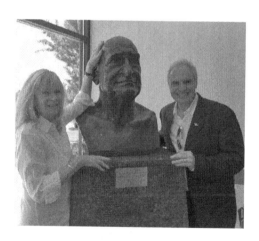

Evelyn and Bob Tarantino, with bust of Reggie

Dear Irene Gold,

I am writing to give you my heartfelt gratitude to you for helping me pass my Part III and Part IV national board exams.

For the record, I took Part III five times with help of a different group before I came to your group, and passed with a 491. My highest previous score on Part III was a 350. Furthermore, I attempted the Part IV exam three times unsuccessfully, also while trying other NB review groups, before finally taking your review course and then passing it.

I want you to understand that I truly appreciate the fact you stayed with me personally for extra-long hours to assure my passing results. I will forever be thankful to you, and without reservation recommend you to every Chiropractor and Chiropractic student who has to complete the national board exam requirements. I know that if you can help me pass these tests, you can help anyone.

Thank you,

T.L.

Dear Reggie,

Your ability to inspire, which is done with unmatched passion, is just one of the many reasons that you are such a giant in Chiropractic. Not everyone may 'get' your message, but nobody can help being touched by the way you deliver it. You do so with love, and because of that I believe your acceptance level is exponentially higher than those who do so in other ways. Personally, you have influenced me on many levels, and my children as well, as my whole family (practice members included) have all benefited from the way the philosophy you've shared has affected me.

You're an amazing man, teacher and Chiropractor, and I feel honored to know you. I had the privilege of sitting with you and Irene at the last New Beginnings during the pre-Halloween party, as well as hearing you speak that weekend, and it is a memory I will cherish for years to come.

With much love, respect and admiration,

John C. D'Ambrosio

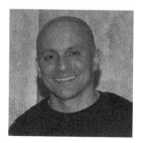

John C. D'Ambrosio

I have just returned from California after taking your wonderful review class for Part III of the national board. I was unable to express my departing words of thanks and my goodbyes to you, as you were at the time inundated with a host of other thankful students expressing to you the same sentiments that I felt. I was also too ill to fight the crowds to get a final hug from you before you left, and I didn't think you would appreciate a hug at that time anyway.

So I am taking the time now to email you, without the flu germs, my sincere sentiments of appreciation for all your kind help for all of us who have nowhere else to turn to get the important information to pass these difficult board exams.

Even though you have a battery of scholarly teachers to assist you when you can't be in all the places at the same time, I now know that no one else can ever fill the shoes of Irene Gold! No one else teaches like you, and no one else commands the attention or the enthusiasm that you provide whenever you teach. Mundane you are not! You are a pure joy to be with and I cannot thank you enough Irene for all your kind, thoughtful efforts and help.

No wonder so many of the students have their picture taken with you, as it provides a cherished keep sake of substantial future proof that they were once fortunate enough to have been a student of the esteemed Dr. Irene Gold. You will go down in Chiropractic history my dear, as an icon to our profession. In my book you are the queen of Chiropractic.

My sincerest, heartfelt thanks to you, and my ultimate respect. You are one dynamic woman. I send this note of appreciation along with the warmest of love and kind thoughts and wishes to you wherever you may go. You are my hero Irene! Thanks for being there when you are so greatly needed.

Eternally thankful, sincerely,

Dr. Gary V. Humphrey

Winter Haven, Florida

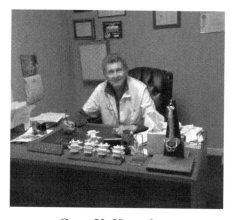

Gary V. Humphrey

Dear Irene,

I just wanted to say thanks for the great review this past month in Tampa. I have to admit that I was extremely nervous about taking this test, and even being able to get through the review. I graduated in October, 1996, so I knew I had my work cut out for me. After the first week of the review I was able to see that not only that I could keep up with everyone, but I was also becoming more relaxed just from the way that you, Dr. Donofrio, and Dr. Kelly explained everything.

Answers came to me quickly and I was able to actually make sense of the things that the examiners wanted for the Florida test. I walked into each portion of the test a little nervous, but confident, and well prepared thanks to you and your team. I kept hearing both John and you in my head saying "one more step."

I really want to tell you that I was so impressed with the way you seem to really care about how each and every one of us did on an individual basis. Offering to get up at 4 or 5 in the morning and being readily available in this day and age is unheard of. I feel completely confident that I passed each part of the examination. I know I put a lot of time in (12 hours a day) but I couldn't have done it without you guys!

Thanks again,

Dean Mammales, DC

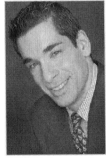

Dean Mammales

Reggie, over 20 years ago you bought my husband and I dinner at the Olive Garden in Davenport, Iowa. You were speaking to our philosophy group at the time. I treasured that dinner. I remember my dad (Dr. Fred Barge) telling me "Now you sit down and listen to that man!" Thanks for all you do Reggie!

Best wishes, love,

Patty

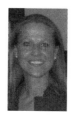

Patty Barge

Hi,

I took the Part I boards for the 4th time in September, 2007, and finally on October 19, 2007, I found out I passed!!! You have no idea the level of confidence I had entering the exams and days later, I never even questioned my performance.

I am very grateful that I decided to take your reviews in Iowa. I am from Chicago, and I attended National University of Health Sciences. I graduated in August of 2007 and still was unable to get through Park I boards. I was going to give up until someone told me about your reviews, and I thought to myself, "oh great, another way for me to spend time and money on something that's probably not going to help."

I had taken reviews in the past, and I bought all the books and material that was out there. I can't thank you enough for offering these reviews, they saved me! I can't wait to take the reviews for Parts II and III.

Kind Regards,

Dr. Evan

Dear Dr. Gold,

Please allow this is to serve as a testimonial of your course:

I graduated from Chiropractic school almost 20 years ago and felt very uncertain about how and what to study for Part IV boards. My concerns faded away with the quality of instruction taught by Dr. Gold and her other instructors. The course sequentially covered the relevant information I needed to know for Part IV, allowing me to have confidence when I took the test. My Part IV results (score 715) are a reflection of Dr. Gold's thoroughness and dedication to the profession. The cost of the course is the best bargain you will find in Chiropractic.

Sincerely,

Fred G. Arnold, DC

Richland Hills, TX

Fred Arnold

Hi Reggie,

I have to say you have always been a Chiropractic "dad" to me. I would bring your 8mm movie in to High School Biology class every year. I loved arguing with everyone about the drugs they were taking and telling them the Chiropractic story. I remember listening to and being inspired by the record of "Valley of the Blind".

My earliest memory of you was when I was in 6th grade. I was at Girl Scout camp in Harriman, NY. I had bad ear infections that summer and my dad came up every few days to give me an adjustment. That kept me in camp until the last few days, when I developed a fever. On the way home, we stopped by your office. I remember the gold wall paper, the fish tank in the wall, and the purple flowered adjusting tables.

My dad has always been a big one for recording things. I had one of his cassettes from an old DE. You were on one side of the tape and Bob Sottile on the other. Both of you were a big influence in my life. I grew up with you as such a strong influence on my dad and thus my philosophy. DE and all the great Chiropractors there, who were so passionate about Chiropractic, has also been an incredible influence in my life. Both are part of my Chiropractic DNA. As such, I never quite understood the schism between the two schools of thought until I heard that tape and the very different message you both spoke. That was enlightening. I still believe that we waste precious time, energy & resources denigrating our brothers that could be better spent changing the world.

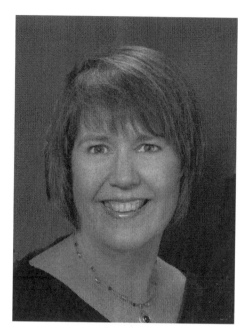

Kim R. Stetzel

Dad recalled lots of stories about the meetings at your house. He remembered being at your office with Bruce Merritt the day you got the call from Lyle Sherman about starting the college. They both wish you their best.

I credit your vision as being the foundation of the family wellness movement in Chiropractic. It was your philosophy which really helped us see that being free of subluxation allows us to express our fullest potential as a human being and that everyone is better off as a clear expression of innate. What a wonderful message to bring to the world.

We are getting set to send a third generation to Chiropractic school, both kids, to carry on the legacy of so many great Chiropractors like you, my dad, Bruce, and countless others. I thank you and Irene for your unswerving commitment to Chiropractic and I wish you both peace.

With love,

Kim R. Stetzel, DC

Hi Irene,

I just completed the x-ray test here in Florida and wanted to send you and Dr. John Donofrio a thank you letter. So thank you.

Irene I know I mentioned to you after the clinical review that I thought your review was outstanding. Not just the preparation of the test, but for all you covered and how you really helped me to understand how the body works. As you know I have been in practice for over 23 years and always felt my clinical to be a weak spot. I'm a great adjusting doctor, I really care for people, and understand the philosophy and that has created success for me. But clinically I was weak, figuring I never really learned the first time around. So thank you for that. I won't shy away from the patients that are a bit confusing to me any longer, so that is a good thing.

Also I have to comment on your enthusiasm, passion and commitment, the way you would hang out at the pool after class and help was fantastic. And the night before our exam how you gave a "heads up" on mitral valve prolapse and that was our test, you are just incredible.

So I have enjoyed going through national boards Parts I-III, and Florida State reviews, and want to thank you for all your help, not just getting me through the tests, but for all that I learned.

Dr. John, thanks to you I got a 91% percent on the Florida test, but more importantly, I now know how to read an x-ray, a good thing for a doctor in practice. Thank you for your help as well, you have the sanest system for reading x-rays that I have ever seen, and I look forward to joining you at the Y Files.

Dr. David

Dear Irene,

You may not remember this brief encounter, but I want to share with you a wonderful visit my wife and I had with you and Reggie.

It was the early 1990s at the Copley Plaza hotel during an ICPA convention. My wife Doreen and I walked in to a nearly empty restaurant and were about to sit for breakfast when we saw you and Reggie having breakfast.

I recall how you were both so friendly and kind as you invited us to join you. We had a wonderful visit. On first impression, you seemed to me to be an unmatched pair, but what I saw that morning were two people who truly enjoyed each other and who were very much in love.

In a world where our leaders are held up as superstars, unapproachable, Reggie was different. He was down to earth and very approachable. He was one of a kind, a real class act. Thank you for sharing him with us and thank you for all the passion you have given to us and this great profession.

God bless you,

Ron Castellucci

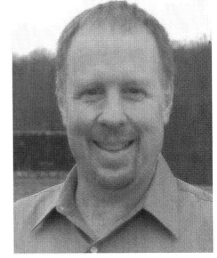

Ron Castellucci

Dear Reggie,

You sat in the front row at the Sherman Lyceum when I spoke there in 2006. I acknowledged you there as the reason for my philosophical clarity and success. I listened to hours and hours of your lectures (on reel to reel) before I got to Chiropractic school. We listened to you through school and it gave me more clarity.

Your message helped Vikki and I build a large family practice in Melbourne. Your message and inspiration helped me become a college president for 8 years, and helped build what is the most focused, congruent Chiropractic college in the world today.

You travelled every year down to the New Zealand Lyceum and helped shape Chiropractic in New Zealand. Your contribution to humanity, to getting more families under care, is unparalleled. We are with you and Irene at this time.

I love you and your unswerving commitment. Thank you my friend.

Dr. Brian D. Kelly, President

Life Chiropractic College West

Hayward, CA

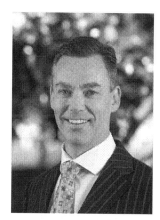

Brian D. Kelly

My Journey into Chiropractic with Reggie Gold:

I had been a loyal Chiropractic "patient" throughout my younger life. Chiropractic saved my mobility after a football injury where my hip was dislocated. After declining a pin in my hip, I was told I would have a limp the rest of my life. After six weeks of Chiropractic care following the injury, I'm still waiting for that limp 63 years later. Chiropractic had also saved me from other problems, too. For all of that, and the rest of my life, I thank my dear mother who had the insight to take me to my first Chiropractor at age 3, in 1947. The Chiropractor named Wilbur Fields had been an MD and returned to Chiropractic school to become a DC. He fixed me in short order.

By a fluke I ended up going to the National College of Chiropractic, having graduated in 1967. After kicking around California for two years, I returned home to the Detroit area to start up my own Chiropractic office. My dad purchased a Chiropractic office from a retiring Palmer doc who did HIO. I had no idea what HIO was, and that started me on a whole new path in life. However, after a year of little traffic through my office, and serious stress headaches daily, I got a call from a local Chiropractor who had seen a lousy little ad I placed in the newspaper entitled "The Eight Danger Signals". I'm glad they called because I had not received any others from my ad.

The local DC called and invited me to a get together with other Chiropractors at his house. As I attended the party, I got the message that it was recruitment for Dynamic Essentials. I decided that I had to go.

At my first DE, I discovered a number of interesting topics and speakers, but the one speaker that stood out was Reggie Gold. After his talk I realized that I had more confidence and belief in Chiropractic prior to going to National College than I did afterwards. Reggie was the Moses to lead me to the promised land.

I would wake up in the middle of the night and have words pouring out of my brain – Chiropractic philosophy. I lost a lot of sleep that way for the first six months after my first DE meeting. The more sleep I lost, the more my practice grew. Within a year I was seeing 150-180 patients per day. (Actually I prefer the term "practice members" ala NSA).

For the next 2-3 years, I followed Reggie to the ends of the earth. After seeing me so often he asked me: "Gary, why do you keep following me around? Ah, I know! Because you love to warm your hands by the fire!" Amen to that, Reg.

After Reggie and Sid Williams parted company, I continued to follow Reggie for a while. I attended one of his monthly gatherings at his home in Spring Valley, NY. I had a PACE (Patients Association for Chiropractic Education) group in my office, and yes, we marched on the Michigan state capitol and did lots of other crazy things. But it was actions such as that the put Chiropractic on the map.

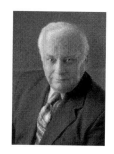

Gary E. Erkfritz

Reggie was in the process of helping Sherman College get started. Then he went on to other things, as did I. But here I am, coming up on my 46th year of practice, now "retired IN practice", and still loving helping people. I thank God every day that Reggie changed my path forever!

Reggie, I'm sure Universal Intelligence has a special place for you – you'll NEVER be forgotten. Thanks for the memories – and the inspiration!

Gary E. Erkfritz, DC

Thousand Oaks, CA

www.drgarye.com

Hi Irene,

I just wanted to write and say thank you so much for your class. I looked at my score last night, I got a 472 on Part III. I never could have done it without your class and your awesome teaching ability. I want to send you a thousand thanks. That was, I think, the 5th time I took the test. You gave me the tools to know how to pick the answers they were looking for. I would recommend your class to anyone. You definitely have the best review class around.

Thanks again and have a great day!

Dr. Chris

Dear Irene,

Thank you for your dedication to ChiropracTIC. Your guidance was crucial in my development as a Chiropractor. You continue to share your blessings with the world and we are all better off because of it.

Much Love and Appreciation,

ADIO y ADIOS,

Liam P. Schübel, DC

Founder of Schübel Vision Worldwide

Founding member of Schübel Vision Seminars

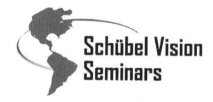

www.schubelvision.com

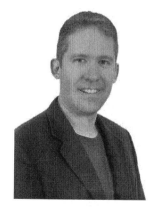

Liam P. Schübel

My Reggie Gold story began 44 years ago. I was 12 years old and I had no idea who Reggie Gold was, but he touched my life and that of my family forever. I had severe stomach aches, pains and other less polite intestinal symptoms. I had all manner of allergies, chocolate, feathers, pollen and whatever else there was. I also had major skin eruptions, acne on my neck and upper torso which was both painful and ugly. But, as I recall, it was the stomach ulcer that put my mother over the top when it came to our health care.

During my 12th year I had been diagnosed using what was called a barium swallow, which is an upper G.I. contrast study of my stomach and esophagus with a fluoroscope. It was determined that I had an ulcer. That was where my stomach pain and symptoms were coming from. Over the course of many months I was given a variety of drugs and diet changes all of which had little or no effect on my pain and were absolutely of no use to my healing. After many months and another upper G.I. series the medics determined that my ulcer had not changed at all. To their credit, they said that the drugs and diet changes had done nothing, but their determination was that, "Your son must just be an uptight kid. He needs to learn how to calm down."

That was my mom's end point. She knew I wasn't uptight, except for not being able to eat. Her lifelong friend worked for a Chiropractor. I'm sure that "aunt Eileen" as we called her, had been suggesting to my mother that we all, especially me, needed to be under Chiropractic care. So, my mom decided that we should go see this Chiropractor, Bruce Merritt.

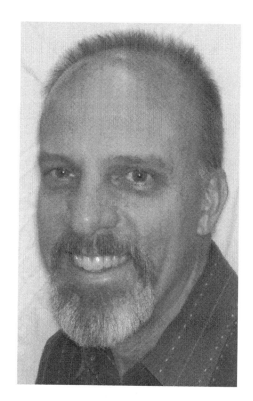

Gary Stewart

The first thing he did was to send home an LP record (you know, one of those black vinyl discs that are about 12 or so inches in diameter) which would explain Chiropractic. As my mother told me, "we are supposed to listen to this record before we can go to his office." Well, before we even listened I was sold on the idea that this kind of doctor did not give drugs or medicine of any kind. I was ready to go. But mom, who always knows best, said we have to listen. So we listened, and I was sold even more. I did not need to hear any more, I knew in my heart that this thing called Chiropractic was right.

It has been over 44 years since that time, I have never been away from Chiropractic care since. I still remember that very first time I heard the Chiropractic principle and philosophy, and the feeling I had in my gut that it is right.

I did not pay any attention at the time to who the speaker on the record was, but I found out later on, as time went by and I became a Chiropractor myself, that it was none other than the great Reggie Gold. I am blessed and fortunate to be able to say that I did have a number of opportunities to meet Reggie, to listen to him live, and to get to know who he was just a little bit better. I also am very grateful for the fact that I now have in my possession one of those records. I believe you said it Reggie, the principle never changes, people change. Fads change, but the principles upon which Chiropractic is founded do not change. So true.

Thank You Reggie!

Gary C. Stewart, Chiropractor

Riverdale, NJ

Dr. Gold,

I walked out of the first part of Part III saying to myself "THANK YOU IRENE GOLD!!!" over and over again. I did so well on Part III, and I credit all that success to you. I cannot thank you enough for all the help you have given me through boards.

My mom was attending National in the 1980s and she was having a hard time passing her first set of boards. National made her stop her curriculum when she didn't pass it the second time. I believe she went down to Iowa and took an Irene Gold review class with her other classmate who was in a similar situation. She passed with flying colors after your review.

Since she had to take time out of school to go and take the review in a different state, she ended up coming back to National and meeting my dad who was a few trimesters behind. All throughout my childhood she would go on and on about Irene Gold and how it helped her pass her boards, become a Chiropractor, and meet my father. Not to sound corny, but I don't think I would even be here if it wasn't for your reviews helping her get through boards and going back to school and meeting my dad!

I really appreciate all you have done for me and my family.

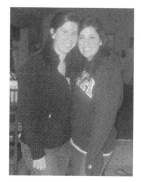

Thanks, Dr. Gold!!

Jaclyn Debs

Jaclyn Debs and her sister Stephanie

Dear Irene,

Thank you so much, for so much! Three things come to mind right now that I need to thank you for.

One, your help in board review. It was not just a refresher cram course to pass the exams, it was much more than that. I actually learned a lot of stuff that I wasn't taught in school, and the stuff I was taught in school, you made easier to actually remember. I passed on the first try, thank you very much.

The second thing was actually during your review course. Somehow you heard I was taking the Neurology Diplomate course and you said, Why do you want to do that? I said to learn more about the core of how our body works, neurology, so I can be a better informed Chiropractor. To which you said, Buy Reggie's tapes, you'll learn more. To which I said, I've listened to them all. To which you said, Then listen to them again!!!!!!!! I LOVED IT!!!!!

Last but not least, thank you for Reggie. It's been said that behind every great man is a great women! I like to think that alongside him, there was you. I'm sure no matter what Reg may have tried to say, he knew that you were an integral part of the legend of "Reggie Gold".

It has been such an honor to have gotten to know you guys on a personal level through the years, and it was so nice seeing you two together at New Beginnings in recent years. He is missed! It is also pretty neat to know that my dad, Jack, shared time with you guys at your office in Spring Valley in his early years. I know it influenced him and therefore influenced me. You never know how far reaching.....

Thanks again Irene.

Love Ya!

Gary DiBenedetto

DC, DACAN, LCP, DPhCS, PhC (Hon), FIACN

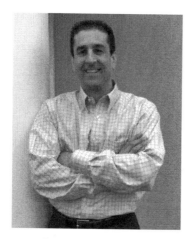

Gary DiBenedetto

Thanks are due to Irene for bringing Chiropractic to the millions of lives she has touched in her many roles in the profession.

Because of Irene, Chiropractors have been produced, careers have been saved, and the Chiropractic message has been delivered on a grand scale. Irene may never see or hear from the patients of her students who have led those people to a higher state of well-being. Yet because of her, the world is a better place.

As B.J. Palmer wrote, "We never know how far reaching something we may think, say, or do today will affect the lives of millions tomorrow."

Christopher Kent

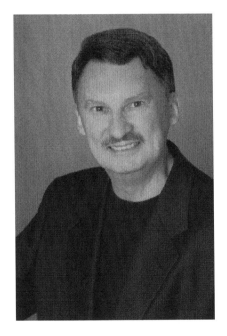

Christopher Kent

Dearest Irene,

I remember the first time I met you. Peter wanted to get your approval of me before he married me...we had dinner with you and Reggie in Sheepshead Bay!! Reggie grilled me about philosophy and you just smiled!! Thank God you approved or I probably wouldn't be married to the most wonderful man on the planet!!!

I love you for all the amazing support and inspiration you have given to me and to so many of my friends in Chiropractic. I love you for all your perseverance, determination, ability, and chutzpah to get the academically challenged minds in our profession to pass the boards. I love you for your humility and graciousness (New York style, of course), and the way you move mountains with your unswerving inner power and resilience.

As I think back to the day that Sigafoose first told me I reminded him of you...it brings tears to my eyes...I don't think I could ever fill your shoes...and if there is a spark of you that he sees in me...I feel blessed and honored.

You are my heroine,

Love, Patti Giuliano, DC

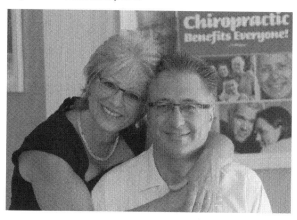

Patti and Peter Giuliano

Dear Reggie,

Thank you so very much for everything that you have given to me. You have given much Chiropractically, but the greatest gift you have added to my life is the example that one's life should be a statement of his or her beliefs, and what it means to think through one's purpose in life and make a full commitment to that purpose. You have been a great leader and beneficiary of the profession. I am sure that few people know of just how generous you and Irene have been to this profession, but I tell them at every opportunity.

Thank you for your great generosity to Sherman College. I believe that it will get back to centering on the vertebral subluxation. I see that we have changed the framing of the Chiropractic problem and with that framing, there is a good possibility that the problem will be properly resolved. This new generation of Chiropractors has many among it who are getting closer to the Big Idea you have spent your life espousing.

Thank you for all you have done for me personally, and especially for the profession.

With great love, appreciation and admiration,

Thom Gelardi

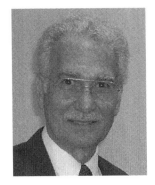

Thom Gelardi

Straight Chiropractors practice Chiropractic because:

- The vertebral subluxation damages all aspects of health, and limits human potential.

- Every man, woman and child should be checked and adjusted if necessary by a Chiropractor.

- Every newborn should have their spine, especially the upper cervical area, checked and adjusted if necessary, within hours after birth, within minutes if possible.

- The Chiropractic adjustment has a pre- and post-analysis that is independent of how a person feels.

- People should have the freedom not to use drugs if they choose.

- Chiropractic should be separate and distinct from the practice of medicine.

- Chiropractic colleges should teach the science, art and philosophy of Chiropractic as their main focus.

- Every student in a Chiropractic college should be taught to analyze the spine for subluxation using the recognized technique of their choice.

Judd Nogrady

Dr. Judd had his life saved and his health restored by Chiropractic care. He now enjoys seeing his practice members achieve a more optimal life and health by maintaining their spines subluxation-free. He takes care of people of all ages at his home practice in Montgomery, NY, as well as his satellite practice in Monroe, NY.

He is the author of an inspirational book entitled "Cast to be Chiropractors." Dr. Judd is also a sought after speaker in the Chiropractic profession. He speaks on many stages around the world and is a founding member of Schübel Vision Seminars, and can be reached at judd1234@frontiernet.net.

He lives with his wife Veronica and his two children, Montana and Jacob, on their organic farm, where they have received national acclaim for their spinach and other organic produce.

Founding member of Schübel Vision Seminars.

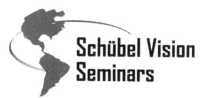

www.schubelvision.com

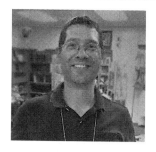

Judd Nogrady

Irene Gold

Irene Gold is currently living in Boca Raton, FL. She is surrounded by her family, and she continues to teach review classes as well as provide private tutoring when necessary.

She can be reached at irenegolddc@aol.com.

Her website is www.irenegoldassoc.com.

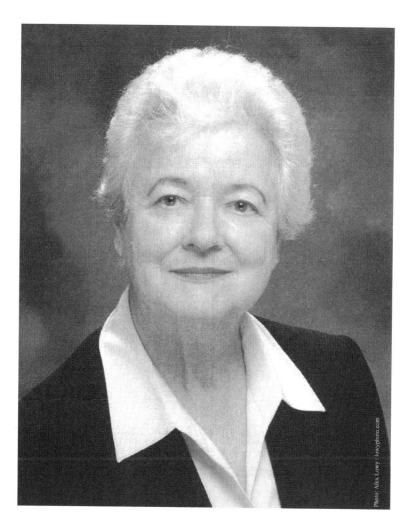

Irene Gold

Made in the USA
Charleston, SC
07 January 2014